Managing the Side Effects of
CHEMOTHERAPY
and
RADIATION

Managing the Side Effects of
CHEMOTHERAPY
and
RADIATION

MARYLIN J. DODD
R.N., Ph.D.

PRENTICE
HALL
PRESS

New York   London   Toronto   Sydney   Tokyo   Singapore

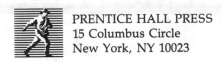

PRENTICE HALL PRESS
15 Columbus Circle
New York, NY 10023

Copyright © 1987 by Appleton & Lange

PRENTICE HALL PRESS and colophon are registered trademarks of
Simon & Schuster, Inc.

Library of Congress Cataloging-in-Publication Data

Dodd, Marylin J.
    Managing the side effects of chemotherapy and radiation /
Marylin J. Dodd.
        p.   cm.
    Includes bibliographical references.
    ISBN 0-13-547480-9
    1. Cancer—Chemotherapy—Complications and sequelae—
Treatment.   2. Cancer—Radiotherapy—Complications and
sequelae—Treatment.   3. Antineoplastic agents—Side
effects.   4. Self-care, Health.   I. Title.
    RC271.C5D62   1991
616.99'4061—dc20   90-7149
                                                                          CIP

Designed by Nina D'Amario/Levavi & Levavi

Manufactured in the United States of America

10 9 8 7 6 5 4

First Prentice Hall Press Edition 1991

ACKNOWLEDGMENTS

The author gratefully acknowledges the important contributions made by several very special people: Mary Thomas, project director of "Coping and Self-Care of Cancer Families," a research grant, and oncology clinical nurse specialist at the Veterans' Administration in Palo Alto; Amy Fitzgerald, radiation nurse specialist at Saint Francis Memorial Hospital; Lisa Hammell, registered dietitian at Pacific Presbyterian Medical Center. A special thank you is extended to the hundreds of oncology patients and their families who conscientiously recorded their activities to manage the side effects of cancer treatment.

CONTENTS

INTRODUCTION

This book will help you and your family learn to better cope with the many side effects of cancer chemotherapy and radiation therapy. Side effects are the undesirable secondary effects of a drug or therapy. Oftentimes cancer patients wonder if the cure is worse than the disease. This book will help you and your loved ones get through treatment and to embark on the voyage of recovery.

In my work as an oncology nurse, I realized that there was a need for this sort of book several years ago. At that time, there was no comprehensive yet easy-to-understand source of information on managing the side effects of chemotherapy and radiation therapy. National cancer groups offered publications for patients, but these were limited in the number of chemotherapeutic agents (drugs) presented, and not specific enough in their suggestions on how to manage side effects of chemo or radiation therapy. Because not enough information was available, patients and their families could not be well-informed participants in their own care. The implications for educating patients are obvious. Patients and families must become actively involved in their treatment and know how to adequately care for themselves.

——— HOW THIS BOOK ——— IS ORGANIZED

The book is divided into two major parts: chemotherapy (Part One) and radiation therapy (Part Two). Part Three consists of The Self-Care Behaviors Log and Patient Appointment Worksheet. Parts One and Two describe the given therapy (chemo or radiation). This explanation is followed by a section that lists in alphabetical order the generic (its abbreviation) and trade names of all commonly used drugs. Frequently occurring side effects of each drug are listed in the first column. The second column explains how to recognize the side effect if it occurs.

Chapter Two offers suggestions for managing possible chemotherapy side effects. The material in this section is presented in the following way:

- *Description.* A brief summary of the nature of the side effect.
- *Duration.* How long the side effect usually lasts.
- *Self-Care Measures.* What the patient and the family can do to manage the side effect.
- *Other Measures.* A description of any other procedures or tests you may need if you experience the side effect (for example, frequent blood pressure readings or blood tests).
- *Consult Physician or Nurse If.* Advice on when you should contact a physician or nurse about the side effect. Even non-life–threatening side effects need to be reported if there is an increase in severity or an

increase in duration, because you can become gravely ill.

* *Also See.* A cross-index of side effects that influence other side effects (or signs and symptoms). For example, if you experience nausea, vomiting, or both, you will probably experience decreased appetite as well. You are directed to the information on how to manage with decreased appetite.

Chapter Four includes thirty-four possible radiation side effects. For each side effect, appropriate measures are described in the same manner as the suggestions for managing chemotherapy side effects are explained above.

The information in this book has been collected from the medical and nursing literature and reviewed by medical oncologists, radiologists, oncology clinical nurse specialists, and pharmacists. The material has been tested in a series of studies examining patients' treatment knowledge (Dodd and Mood, 1981; Dodd, 1982a) and self-care activities (Dodd, 1982b, 1983, 1984a, 1984b, 1984c, 1986, 1987, 1988a, 1988b). These studies included patients with many types of cancer, receiving different chemotherapy or radiation therapy. References are provided for the reader who desires more detailed information.

The Self-Care Behaviors Log has been developed and tested to enable you to record the side effects you may experience, the side effects you actually experience, and the activities you undertake to prevent or manage them. You will describe how severe and distressing these side effects are, your actions and their effectiveness, and who provided you with the idea for the self-care activity. This log has been used successfully by many people with cancer.

Because there is a lot to remember, I've also included a Patient Appointment Worksheet (page 199). You can write down the time and date of your next appointment, and questions to ask or things to tell the physician or nurse.

——HOW TO USE THIS BOOK——

1. You need to know the specific chemotherapeutic drugs you are to receive or, in the case of radiation therapy, what part of your body will receive radiation.
2. You should then read the general introduction on chemotherapy (pages 3 to 4).
3. You should then review the chemotherapeutic drugs or the radiation therapy you will receive, and the potential side effects, signs, and symptoms described in the chemotherapy or radiation therapy parts of the book.
4. Finally, you should read the sections on how to record information in the Self-Care Behaviors Log. The first section of the log is preventive. You try to recall the potential side effects of therapy that the physician or nurse has mentioned. These potential side effects are recorded along with any self-care activity you should initiate, possibly with assistance from a family member, to decrease the likelihood of that side effect occurring. If you experience the side effect, you are to record this in the second section of the log, and also to record its severity, distress, and the self-care activities you performed to manage the side effect. Be sure to bring the log to the clinic at each chemo appointment or weekly for the duration of radiation treat-

ment. The log provides the nurse and physician with a record of which side effects you have experienced and the self-care activities you have undertaken. On a continuing basis, the nurse and physician can make suggestions for managing side effects. The record of experienced side effects helps you to remember what has happened since the last clinic appointment, and may help you to overcome the reluctance of telling the nurse or physician what side effects have occurred.

These guidelines on how to use the book are mainly suggestions. Obviously, all information relevant to you regarding chemotherapy or radiation therapy cannot be absorbed at once. This book offers the opportunity to systematically prepare and manage the side effects as they threaten or occur over time.

Some nurses and physicians believe that if patients are given information on the possible side effects of treatment, they become more susceptible to developing these side effects, or the side effects increase in their severity. In the studies referred to earlier, this has not been the case. Patients who received comprehensive treatment information have not reported an increase in experienced side effects and have performed many more self-care activities than patients who did not receive this information (Dodd and Mood, 1981; Dodd, 1982a, 1983, 1984a, 1988a, 1988b).

In summary, this book provides you and your family with useful information on cancer treatment. There is no question that you can more fully participate in your care or the care of a family member who has cancer by reporting, preventing, and managing the side effects of treatment.

PART I

———

Chemotherapy

WHAT IS CHEMOTHERAPY?

Chemotherapy is the use of drugs to destroy cancer cells. Chemotherapeutic drugs affect cells (cancer and normal cells), which accounts for some drug side effects. The side effects from chemotherapy are temporary and subside once the drugs have been discontinued upon completion of treatment. Regrowth of the rapidly dividing normal cells that have been injured sometimes occurs even before the drugs are discontinued, but usually growth begins after the treatment is over. If you experience a side effect from chemotherapy, it does not mean that something is wrong or that the drugs you are taking are not destroying cancer cells. You may or may not experience some of the side effects associated with each individual drug. Each person reacts differently to chemotherapy.

The chemotherapy information presented here was

designed to help you recognize any signs of symptoms you experience during your treatment. By knowing the signs and symptoms of the potential side effects, you can alert your physician or nurse to their occurrence before the side effects become severe.

The chemotherapy part of this book has two sections. The first lists forty-eight common chemotherapeutic drugs and their side effects. The second section offers suggestions for managing each side effect listed. It would be very helpful if your nurse or physician would indicate in this book the drugs you are receiving and the side effects that might occur. Also, it would be helpful if they reviewed your Self-Care Behaviors Log with you during your clinic visits.

——COMMONLY USED DRUGS——

Aminoglutethimide (Cytadren)	Cytarabine [ARA-C] (Cytosar; Cytarabine)
Amsacrine [m-AMSA]	Dacarbazine [DTIC] (DTIC Dome)
5-Azacytidine [5-AC]	
Bleomycin sulfate (Blenoxane)	Dactinomycin (Cosmegen)
Busulfan (Myleran)	Daunorubicin hydrochloride or Daunomycin (Cerubidine)
Carboplatin (Paraplatin)	
Carmustine [BCNU], (BiCNU)	
Chlorambucil (Leukeran)	Dichloromethotrexate [DCMXT]
Chlorozotocin [DCNU]	Diethylstilbestrol [DES]
Cisplatin [DDP] (Platinol)	Doxorubicin hydrochloride (Adriamycin)
Cyclophosphamide ╱ (Cytoxan)	Estrogen
	Etoposide [VP-16]

Floxuridine [FUDR]
✓ Fluorouracil [5-FU]
Flutamide (Eulexin)
Hexamethylmelamine
  [HMM, HXM]
Hydroxyurea (Hydrea)
Ifosfamide (IFEX)
L-Asparaginase (Elspar)
Leuprolide (Lupron)
Lomustine [CCNU]
  (CeeNU)
Maytansine
Mechlorethamine
  hydrochloride
  (Mustargen)
Medroxyprogesterone
  acetate (Provera;
  Depo-Provera)
Megestrol acetate
  (Megace)
Melphalan [L-PAM]
  (Alkeran)
Mercaptopurine [6-MP]

✓ Methotrexate [MTX]
  sodium
Mithramycin or
  Plicamycin (Mithracin)
Mitomycin (Mutamycin)
Mitoxantrone
  hydrochloride
✓ (Novantrone)
Prednisone
Procarbazine
  hydrochloride
  (Matulane)
Streptozocin (Zanosar)
Tamoxifen citrate
  (Nolvadex)
Teniposide [VM-26]
Thioguanine [6-TG]
Thio-tepa (Thiotepa)
Vinblastine sulfate
  (Velban)
✓ Vincristine sulfate
  (Oncovin)

ONE

Possible Side Effects, Signs, and Symptoms

AMINOGLUTETHIMIDE
(Cytadren)

POSSIBLE SIDE EFFECTS	SIGNS AND SYMPTOMS
Skin rash, itching, peeling, hives (dermatitis)	
Tiredness, fatigue	
Blood pressure, decreased (hypotension)	Dizziness, lightheadedness when changing positions and standing
Infection, fewer white blood cells (leukopenia)	Sore throat, cough, stuffy nose; burning when you urinate; shaking chills; diarrhea; burning (pain) when you have a bowel movement; pain, redness, swelling, and heat if you hurt your skin; temperature above 100.5°F (38°C); eyes or ears drain

Nausea and vomit-
ing
Appetite, de-
creased (ano-
rexia)

———— AMSACRINE ————
[m-AMSA]

POSSIBLE SIDE EFFECTS	SIGNS AND SYMPTOMS
Infection, fewer white blood cells (leukopenia)	Sore throat, cough, stuffy nose; burning when you urinate; shaking chills; diarrhea; burning (pain) when you have a bowel movement; pain, redness, swelling, and heat if you hurt your skin; temperature above 100.5°F (38°C); eyes or ears drain
Liver damage, liver poisoning	Yellow skin and yellow tinge to the whites of your eyes; nausea; fatigue; pain on right side
Blood in urine (hematuria)	You need to urinate frequently, but it is difficult to urinate; urine has pink color and maybe some blood clots; low back pain
Hair thinning or loss (alopecia)	Hair on your head and body thins and falls out
Mouth sores (stomatitis)	Mouth, gums, and throat feel sore (raw), burning, or different; red mouth and gums
Nausea and vomiting	
Skin rash, itching, peeling, hives (dermatitis)	
Heart damage	Puffiness or swelling of your hands and ankles; shortness of breath; loss of appetite; skipped heartbeat or palpitations

AZACYTIDINE [5-AC]

POSSIBLE SIDE EFFECTS	SIGNS AND SYMPTOMS
Infection, fewer white blood cells (leukopenia)	Sore throat, cough, stuffy nose; burning when you urinate; shaking chills; diarrhea; burning (pain) when you have a bowel movement; pain, redness, swelling, and heat if you hurt your skin; temperature above 100.5°F (38°C); eyes or ears drain
Bleeding, low platelet count (thrombocytopenia)	Unexplained bruises; bleeding gums; nosebleed; blood in your vomit or stools may be red or black and tarry; blood in urine or sputum; headache, visual changes (loss of a portion of your field of vision or blurriness); increased flow with menses
Anemia, fewer red blood cells	More tired than usual; dizzy when you change positions; lightheadedness; pale membranes (lining) in your mouth and inner eyelids; feel cold more often; insomnia, nervousness
Nausea and vomiting	
Diarrhea	
Liver damage, liver poisoning	Yellow skin and yellow tinge to the whites of your eyes; nausea, fatigue; pain on right side
Fever	
Skin rash, itching, peeling, hives (dermatitis)	
Blood pressure, decreased (hypotension)	Dizziness, lightheadedness when changing positions and standing
Muscle pain	

Muscle weakness

Mouth sores (sto-matitis)	Mouth, gums, and throat feel sore (raw), burning, or different, red mouth and gums

——— BLEOMYCIN SULFATE ———
(Blenoxane)

POSSIBLE SIDE EFFECTS	SIGNS AND SYMPTOMS
Fever	
Blood pressure, low (hypoten-sion)	Dizziness, lightheadedness when changing positions and standing
Nausea and vomit-ing	
Skin rash, itching, peeling, hives (dermatitis)	
Mouth sores (sto-matitis)	Mouth, gums, and throat may feel sore (raw), burning, or different; red-dened areas in mouth and on gums
Pain at the site where you were given your che-motherapy or near your tumor soon after you take your che-motherapy drug(s)	
Hair, thinning or loss (alopecia)	Hair on your head and body thins and falls out

Shortness of breath, dry cough (dyspnea; pulmonary fibrosis)	Occurs when you walk fast, climb stairs, or work physically
Allergic reaction after chemotherapy (hypersensitivity)	Fever and chills occurring within 3 to 6 hours after chemotherapy was given; notify nurse or physician immediately

——— BUSULFAN (Myleran) ———

POSSIBLE SIDE EFFECTS	SIGNS AND SYMPTOMS
Fever	
Appetite, decreased (anorexia)	
Shortness of breath, dry cough (dyspnea; pulmonary fibrosis)	Occurs when you walk fast, climb stairs, or do hard work
Skin is darker (hyperpigmentation)	Creases on skin of your hands
Menstrual periods are irregular (amenorrhea)	Some women stop monthly menstrual cycle but can still become pregnant
Sexual dysfunction, sterility	Impotence and decreased libido, menstrual irregularities, adverse effects on fetal development (if conception occurs, drug adversely impacts the reproductive system)

Infection, fewer white blood cells (leukopenia)	Sore throat, cough, stuffy nose; burning when you urinate; shaking chills; diarrhea; burning (pain) when you have a bowel movement; pain, redness, swelling, and heat if you hurt your skin; temperature above 100.5°F (38°C); eyes or ears drain
Bleeding, low platelet count (thrombocytopenia)	Bruises, bleeding gums; nosebleeds; blood in your vomit may be bright red or coffee-ground-like; blood in stool may be red or black and tarry; blood in urine or sputum; headache; visual changes (loss of a portion of your field of vision or blurriness); increased flow with menses

——— CARBOPLATIN (Paraplatin) ———

POSSIBLE SIDE EFFECTS	SIGNS AND SYMPTOMS
Nausea and vomiting	
Bleeding, low platelet count (thrombocytopenia)	Unexplained bruises; bleeding gums; nosebleeds; blood in your vomit may be red or black and tarry; blood in urine or sputum; headache; visual changes (loss of a portion of your field of vision or blurriness); increased flow with menses
Infection, fewer white blood cells (leukopenia)	Sore throat, cough, stuffy nose; burning when you urinate; shaking chills; diarrhea; burning (pain) when you have a bowel movement; pain, redness, swelling, and heat if you hurt your skin; temperature above 100.5°F (38°C); eyes and ears drain

Anemia, fewer red blood cells	More tired than usual; dizzy when you change positions; lightheadedness; pale membranes (lining) in your mouth and inner eyelids; feel cold more often; insomnia; feeling nervous
Numbness, tingling in hands and feet (peripheral neuropathies)	Clumsiness of hands and feet; feeling of weakness in fingers and toes; feeling a different sensation in fingers and toes

——— CARMUSTINE [BCNU] (BiCNU) ———

POSSIBLE SIDE EFFECTS	SIGNS AND SYMPTOMS
Pain or burning at the site where you were given your chemotherapy or near your tumor soon after you take your chemotherapy drug(s)	
Nausea and vomiting	
Infection, fewer white blood cells (leukopenia)	Sore throat, cough, stuffy nose; burning when you urinate; shaking chills; diarrhea; burning (pain) when you have a bowel movement; pain, redness, swelling, and heat if you hurt your skin; temperature above 100.5°F (38°C); eyes or ears drain
Bleeding, low platelet count (thrombocytopenia)	Unexplained bruises; bleeding gums; nosebleeds; blood in your vomit may be bright red or coffee-ground-like; blood in stool may be red or black and tarry; blood in urine or sputum; headache; visual changes (loss of a portion of your field of vision or blurriness); increased flow with menses

Liver damage, liver poisoning

Yellow skin and yellow tinge to the whites of your eyes; nausea; fatigue; pain on right side

Kidney damage, kidney poisoning

Headache; puffiness at the ankles and hands; flank pain

Shortness of breath, dry cough (dyspnea; pulmonary fibrosis)

Occurs when you walk fast, climb stairs, or do hard work

Blood pressure, decreased (hypotension)

Dizziness; lightheadedness when changing positions and standing

Mouth sores (stomatitis)

Mouth, gums, and throat may feel sore (raw), burning, or different; reddened areas in mouth and on gums

——— CHLORAMBUCIL (Leukeran) ———

POSSIBLE SIDE EFFECTS

SIGNS AND SYMPTOMS

Infection, fewer white blood cells (leukopenia)

Sore throat, cough, stuffy nose; burning when you urinate; shaking chills; diarrhea; burning (pain) when you have a bowel movement; pain, redness, swelling, and heat if

you hurt your skin; temperature above 100.5°F (38°C); eyes or ears drain

Bleeding, low platelet count (thrombocytopenia)

Unexplained bruises; bleeding gums; nosebleeds; blood in your vomit may be bright red or coffee-ground-like; blood in stool may be red or black and tarry; blood in urine or sputum; headache; visual changes (loss of a portion of your field of vision or blurriness); increased flow with menses

Nausea and vomiting

Liver damage, liver poisoning	Yellow skin and yellow tinge to the whites of your eyes; nausea; fatigue; pain on right side
Sexual dysfunction, sterility	Impotence and decreased libido, menstrual irregularities, adverse effects on fetal development (if conception occurs, drug adversely impacts the reproductive system)
Anemia, fewer red blood cells	More tired than usual; dizzy when you change positions; lightheadedness; pale membranes (lining) in your mouth and inner eyelids; feel cold more often; insomnia; nervousness

———— CHLOROZOTOCIN [DCNU] ————

POSSIBLE SIDE EFFECTS	SIGNS AND SYMPTOMS
Nausea and vomiting	
Liver damage, liver poisoning	Yellow skin and yellow tinge to the whites of your eyes; nausea; fatigue; pain on right side
Infection, fewer white blood cells (leukopenia)	Sore throat, cough, stuffy nose; burning when you urinate; shaking chills; diarrhea; burning (pain) when you have a bowel movement; pain, redness, swelling, and heat if you hurt your skin; temperature above 100.5°F (38°C); eyes or ears drain
Bleeding, low platelet count (thrombocytopenia)	Unexplained bruises; bleeding gums; nosebleeds; blood in your vomit may be bright red or coffee-ground-like; blood in stool may be red or black and tarry; blood in urine or sputum; headache; visual changes (loss of a portion of your field of vision or blurriness); increased flow with menses

———— CISPLATIN [DDP] (Platinol) ————

POSSIBLE SIDE EFFECTS	SIGNS AND SYMPTOMS
Ringing in your ears (tinnitus)	
Hearing loss (ototoxicity)	Inability to hear normal or usual noise tones; notify nurse or physician immediately
Nausea and vomiting	
Liver damage, liver poisoning	Yellow skin and yellow tinge to the whites of your eyes; nausea; fatigue; pain on right side
Kidney damage, kidney poisoning	Headache; puffiness at the ankles and hands; flank pain
Infection, fewer white blood cells (leukopenia)	Sore throat, cough, stuffy nose; burning when you urinate; shaking chills; diarrhea; burning (pain) when you have a bowel movement; pain, redness, swelling, and heat if you hurt your skin; temperature above 100.5°F (38°C); eyes or ears drain
Bleeding, low platelet count (thrombocytopenia)	Unexplained bruises; bleeding gums; nosebleeds; blood in your vomit may be bright red or coffee-ground-like; blood in stool may be red or black and tarry; blood in urine or sputum; headache; visual changes (loss of a portion of your field of vision or blurriness); increased flow with menses
Allergic reaction immediately after chemotherapy (hypersensitivity)	Fast heartbeat, wheezing, lightheadedness when moving; notify nurse or physician immediately

Anemia, fewer red blood cells	More tired than usual; dizzy when you change positions; lightheadedness; pale membranes (lining) in your mouth and inner eyelids; feel cold more often; insomnia; nervousness
Numbness, tingling in hands and feet (peripheral neuropathies)	Clumsiness in hands and feet and/or they feel different to you, different sensation
Skin burning as needle delivering chemotherapy comes out of the vein (extravasation)	Swelling, redness, warmth, and pain over skin, notify the physician or nurse immediately
Taste changes	

———— CYCLOPHOSPHAMIDE ————
(Cytoxan)

POSSIBLE SIDE EFFECTS	SIGNS AND SYMPTOMS
Nausea and vomiting	
Infection, fewer white blood cells (leukopenia)	Sore throat, cough, stuffy nose; burning when you urinate; shaking chills; diarrhea; burning (pain) when you have a bowel movement; pain, redness, swelling, and heat if you hurt your skin; temperature above 100.5°F (38°C); eyes or ears drain
Pigmentation, increased coloring of the skin and fingernails	

Bleeding, low platelet count (thrombocytopenia)	Unexplained bruises; bleeding gums; nosebleeds; blood in your vomit may be bright red or coffee-ground-like; blood in stool may be red or black and tarry; blood in urine or sputum; headache; visual changes (loss of a portion of your field of vision or blurriness); increased flow with menses
Hair thinning or loss (alopecia)	Hair on your head and body thins and falls out
Blood in urine (hematuria)	You need to urinate frequently, but it is difficult to urinate; urine has pink color and sometimes has blood clots; low back pain
Appetite, decreased (anorexia)	
Sexual dysfunction, sterility	Impotence and decreased libido, menstrual irregularities, adverse effects on fetal development (if conception occurs, drug adversely impacts the reproductive system)
Taste change	Metallic taste in mouth
Anemic, fewer red blood cells	More tired than usual; dizzy when you change positions; lightheadedness; pale membranes (lining) in mouth and eyes; feel cold more often; insomnia; nervousness

——— CYTARABINE [ARA-C] ———
(Cytosar; Cytarabine)

POSSIBLE SIDE EFFECTS	SIGNS AND SYMPTOMS
Nausea and vomiting	
Mouth sores (stomatitis)	Mouth, gums, and throat feel sore (raw), burning, or different; red mouth and gums

Bleeding, low platelet count (thrombocytopenia)	Unexplained bruises; bleeding gums; nosebleeds; blood in your vomit may be bright red or coffee-ground-like; blood in stool may be red or black and tarry; blood in urine or sputum; headache; visual changes (loss of a portion of your field of vision or blurriness); increased flow with menses
Infection, fewer white blood cells (leukopenia)	Sore throat, cough, stuffy nose; burning when you urinate; shaking chills; diarrhea; burning (pain) when you have a bowel movement; pain, redness, swelling, and heat if you hurt your skin; temperature above 100.5°F (38°C); eyes or ears drain
Skin rash, itching, peeling, hives (dermatitis)	
Diarrhea	
Liver damage, liver poisoning	Yellow skin and yellow tinge to the whites of your eyes; nausea; fatigue; pain on right side
Appetite, decreased (anorexia)	
Sexual dysfunction, sterility	Impotence and decreased libido, menstrual irregularities, adverse effects on fetal development (if conception occurs, drug adversely impacts the reproductive system)
Flulike syndrome	Muscle aches; fatigue; nausea; slight oral temperature; loss of appetite

———— DACARBAZINE [DTIC] ————
(DTIC Dome)

POSSIBLE SIDE EFFECTS	SIGNS AND SYMPTOMS
Nausea and vomiting	
Bleeding, low platelet count (thrombocytopenia)	Unexplained bruises; bleeding gums; nosebleeds; blood in your vomit may be red or black and tarry; blood in urine or sputum; headache; visual changes (loss of a portion of your field of vision or blurriness); increased flow with menses
Infection, fewer white blood cells (leukopenia)	Sore throat, cough, stuffy nose; burning when you urinate; shaking chills; diarrhea; burning (pain) when you have a bowel movement; pain, redness, swelling, and heat if you hurt your skin; temperature above 100.5°F (38°C); eyes or ears drain
Flulike syndrome	Muscle aches; fatigue; nausea; slightly raised oral temperature; loss of appetite
Hair, thinning or loss (alopecia)	Hair on your head and/or body thins and falls out
Anemia, fewer red blood cells	More tired than usual; dizzy when you change positions; lightheadedness; pale membranes (lining) in your mouth and eyes; feel cold more often; insomnia; nervousness
Liver damage, liver poisoning	Yellow skin and yellow tinge to the whites of your eyes; nausea; fatigue; pain on right side
Skin, burning if needle delivering chemotherapy is removed from the vein (extravasation)	Swelling, redness, warmth, and pain over the skin; notify the physician or nurse immediately

Appetite, de-
creased (ano-
rexia)

──────── DACTINOMYCIN (Cosmegen) ────────

POSSIBLE SIDE EFFECTS	SIGNS AND SYMPTOMS
Nausea and vomiting	
Appetite, decreased (anorexia)	
Infection, fewer white blood cells (leukopenia)	Sore throat, cough, stuffy nose; burning when you urinate; shaking chills; diarrhea; burning (pain) when you have a bowel movement; pain, redness, swelling, and heat if you hurt your skin; temperature above 100.5°F (38°C); eyes or ears drain
Bleeding, low platelet count (thrombocytopenia)	Unexplained bruises; bleeding gums; nosebleeds; blood in your vomit may be bright red or coffee-ground-like; blood in stool may be red or black and tarry; blood in urine or sputum; headache; visual changes (loss of a portion of your field of vision or blurriness); increased flow with menses
Anemia, fewer red blood cells	More tired than usual; dizzy when you change positions; lightheadedness; pale membranes (lining) in mouth and eyes; feel cold more often; insomnia; nervousness
Pigmentation, increased coloring of the skin	
Hair thinning or loss (alopecia)	Hair on your head and body thins and falls out

Skin changes in areas that have been previously treated with radiation (hyperpigmentation)	Skin becomes red, peels, or becomes darker; acne and rash may appear
Mouth sores (stomatitis)	Mouth, gums, and throat feel sore (raw), burning, or different; red mouth and gums
Skin burning as needle delivering chemotherapy comes out of the vein (extravasation)	Swelling, redness, warmth, and pain over skin; notify the physician or nurse immediately
Diarrhea	

——— DAUNORUBICIN ——— HYDROCHLORIDE (Cerubidine)

POSSIBLE SIDE EFFECTS	SIGNS AND SYMPTOMS
Infection, fewer white blood cells (leukopenia)	Sore throat, cough, stuffy nose; burning when you urinate; shaking chills; diarrhea; burning (pain) when you have a bowel movement; pain, redness, swelling, and heat if you hurt your skin; temperature above 100.5°F (38°C); eyes or ears drain
Bleeding, low platelet count (thrombocytopenia)	Unexplained bruises; bleeding gums; nosebleeds; blood in your vomit may be red or black and tarry; blood in urine or sputum; headache; visual changes (loss of a portion of your field of vision or blurriness); increased flow with menses
Heart damage	Puffiness or swelling of your hands and ankles; short of breath; loss of appetite; skipped heartbeat or palpitations

Skin burning as needle delivering chemotherapy comes out of the vein (extravasation)	Swelling, redness, warmth, and pain over skin; notify the physician or nurse immediately
Red color of urine	Drug is red and temporarily colors the urine
Skin changes in areas that have been previously treated with radiation (hyperpigmentation)	Skin becomes red, peels, or becomes darker; acne and rash may appear
Hair thinning or loss (alopecia)	Hair on your head and body falls out
Nausea and vomiting	
Anemia, low red blood cells	More tired than usual; dizzy when you change positions; lightheadedness; pale membranes (lining) in your mouth and eyes; feel cold more often; insomnia; nervousness
Mouth sores (stomatitis)	Mouth, gums, and throat feel sore (raw), burning, or different; red mouth and gums

——— DICHLOROMETHOTREXATE ——— [DCMXT]

POSSIBLE SIDE EFFECTS	SIGNS AND SYMPTOMS
Nausea and vomiting	
Mouth sores (stomatitis)	Mouth, gums, and throat feel sore (raw), burning, or different; red mouth and gums

Liver damage, liver poisoning	Yellow skin and yellow tinge to the whites of your eyes; nausea; fatigue; pain on right side
Kidney damage, kidney poisoning	Headache; puffiness at the ankles and hands; flank pain
Infection, fewer white blood cells (leukopenia)	Sore throat, cough, stuffy nose; burning when you urinate; shaking chills; diarrhea; burning (pain) when you have a bowel movement; pain, redness, swelling, and heat if you hurt your skin; temperature above 100.5°F (38°C); eyes or ears drain
Bleeding, low platelet count (thrombocytopenia)	Unexplained bruises; bleeding gums; nosebleeds; blood in your vomit may be bright red or coffee-ground-like; blood in stool may be red or black and tarry; blood in urine or sputum; headache; visual changes (loss of a portion of your field of vision or blurriness); increased flow with menses
Anemia, fewer red blood cells	More tired than usual; dizzy when you change positions; lightheadedness; pale membranes (lining) in your mouth and eyes; feel cold more often; insomnia; nervousness
Diarrhea	

——— DIETHYLSTILBESTROL [DES] ———

POSSIBLE SIDE EFFECTS	SIGNS AND SYMPTOMS
Sexual dysfunction, sterility	May cause severe harm to fetus; feminization in men; menstrual irregularities
Nausea and vomiting	
Weight increase with fluid retention (edema)	Puffiness (swelling of your ankles and hands) and overall weight gain

Muscle weakness

Appetite, de-
creased (ano-
rexia)

DOXORUBICIN HYDROCHLORIDE (Adriamycin)

POSSIBLE SIDE EFFECTS	SIGNS AND SYMPTOMS
Nausea and vomiting	
Mouth sores (stomatitis)	Mouth, gums, and throat feel sore (raw), burning, or different; red mouth and gums
Diarrhea	
Hair thinning or loss (alopecia)	Hair on your head and body thins and falls out
Mood changes	Sudden mood changes; you may feel ''blue'' or find yourself crying for no apparent reason
Red color of urine	Drug is red and temporarily colors the urine
Infection, fewer white blood cells (leukopenia)	Sore throat, cough, stuffy nose; burning when you urinate; shaking chills; diarrhea; burning (pain) when you have a bowel movement; pain, redness, swelling, and heat if you hurt your skin; temperature above 100.5°F (38°C); eyes or ears drain
Bleeding, low platelet count (thrombocytopenia)	Unexplained bruises; bleeding gums; nosebleeds; blood in your vomit may be bright red or coffee-ground-like; blood in stool may be red or black and tarry; blood in urine or sputum; headache; visual changes (loss of a portion of your field of vision or blurriness); increased flow with menses

Possible Side Effects, Signs, and Symptoms

Heart damage	Puffiness or swelling of your hands and ankles; short of breath; loss of appetite; skipped heartbeat or palpitations
Anemia, fewer red blood cells	More tired than usual; dizzy when you change positions; lightheadedness; pale membranes (lining) in your mouth and eyes; feel cold more often; insomnia; nervousness
Skin, burning as needle delivering chemotherapy comes out of the vein (extravasation)	Swelling, redness, warmth, and pain over skin; notify the physician or nurse immediately
Skin changes in areas that have been treated with radiation	Skin becomes red, peels, or becomes darker; acne and rash may appear

——— ESTROGEN ———

POSSIBLE SIDE EFFECTS	SIGNS AND SYMTPOMS
Nausea and vomiting	
Weight increase with fluid retention (edema)	Puffiness (swelling of your ankles and hands) and overall weight gain
Sexual dysfunction (feminization in men, menstrual irregularities)	Enlarged breasts; decreased sexual drive; less and finer body hair
Muscle weakness	
Appetite, decreased (anorexia)	

——— ETOPOSIDE [VP-16] ———

POSSIBLE SIDE EFFECTS	SIGNS AND SYMPTOMS
Anemia, fewer red blood cells	More tired than usual; dizzy when you change positions; lightheadedness; pale membranes (lining) in your mouth and eyes; feel cold more often; insomnia; nervousness
Bleeding, low platelet count (thrombocytopenia)	Unexplained bruises; bleeding gums; nosebleeds; blood in your vomit may be bright red or coffee-ground-like; blood in stool may be red or black and tarry; blood in urine or sputum; headache; visual changes (loss of a portion of your field of vision or blurriness); increased flow with menses
Infection, fewer white blood cells (leukopenia)	Sore throat, cough, stuffy nose; burning when you urinate; shaking chills; diarrhea; burning (pain) when you have a bowel movement; pain, redness, swelling, and heat if you hurt your skin; temperature above 100.5°F (38°C); eyes or ears drain
Nausea and vomiting	
Fever, caused by chemotherapy	
Blood pressure, decreased (hypotension)	Dizziness, light-headedness when changing positions and standing
Hair thinning or loss (alopecia)	Hair in your head and body thins and falls out

Appetite, de-
creased (ano-
rexia)

Allergic reaction im- mediately after chemotherapy (hypersensitivity)	Fast heartbeat, wheezing, lightheaded- ness when moving; notify nurse or physician immediately

——— FLOXURIDE [FUDR] ———

POSSIBLE SIDE EFFECTS	SIGNS AND SYMPTOMS
Nausea and vomit- ing	
Diarrhea	
Infection, fewer white blood cells (leukopenia)	Sore throat, cough, stuffy nose; burn- ing when you urinate; shaking chills; diarrhea; burning (pain) when you have a bowel movement; pain, red- ness, swelling, and heat if you hurt your skin; temperature above 100.5°F (38°C); eyes or ears drain
Bleeding, low plate- let count (throm- bocytopenia)	Unexplained bruises; bleeding gums; nosebleeds; blood in your vomit may be bright red or coffee-ground-like; blood in stool may be red or black and tarry; blood in urine or sputum; head- ache; visual changes (loss of a portion of your field of vision or blurriness); in- crease in flow with menses
Hair thinning or loss (alopecia)	Hair in your head and body thins and falls out
Mouth sores (sto- matitis)	Mouth, gums, and throat feel sore (raw), burning, or different; red mouth and gums
Appetite, de- creased (ano- rexia)	

Abdominal cramps
and pain

Blurred vision, diz-
ziness (vertigo),
tiredness

Anemia, fewer red blood cells	More tired than usual; dizzy when you change positions; lightheadedness; pale membranes (lining) in your mouth and eyes; feel cold more often; insomnia; nervousness
Sexual dysfunc- tion, sterility	Impotence and decreased libido, men- strual irregularities, adverse effects on fetal development (if conception oc- curs, drug adversely impacts the re- productive system)

Skin rash, itching,
peeling (dermati-
tis); pigmenta-
tion may also
increase

———— FLUOROURACIL [5-FU] ————

**POSSIBLE SIDE
EFFECTS**

SIGNS AND SYMPTOMS

Nausea and vomit-
ing

Diarrhea

Infection, fewer white blood cells (leukopenia)	Sore throat, cough, stuffy nose; burn- ing when you urinate; shaking chills; diarrhea; burning (pain) when you have a bowel movement; pain, red- ness, swelling, and heat if you hurt your skin; temperature above 100.5°F (38°C); eyes or ears drain

Bleeding, low platelet count (thrombocytopenia)	Unexplained bruises; bleeding gums; nosebleeds; blood in your vomit may be bright red or coffee-ground-like; blood in stool may be red or black and tarry; blood in urine or sputum; headache; visual changes (loss of a portion of your field of vision or blurriness); increased flow with menses
Hair thinning or loss (alopecia)	Hair on your head and body thins and falls out
Mouth sores (stomatitis)	Mouth, gums, and throat feel sore (raw), burning, or different; red mouth and gums
Appetite, decreased (anorexia)	
Abdominal cramps and pain	
Tiredness	May occur 2 to 3 days after injection; generally stops in 2 to 3 days
Skin rash	May appear on areas exposed to the sun, but rarely requires stopping the drug; the color of your skin and veins may darken
Sexual dysfunction, sterility	Impotence and decreased libido, menstrual irregularities, adverse effects on fetal development (if conception occurs, drug adversely impacts the reproductive system)

———— FLUTAMIDE (Eulexin) ————

POSSIBLE SIDE EFFECTS	SIGNS AND SYMPTOMS
Sexual dysfunction, sterility	Impotence and decreased libido, menstrual irregularities, adverse effects on fetal development (if conception occurs, drug adversely impacts the reproductive system)

Hot flashes
Diarrhea
Nausea and vomit-
ing

——— HEXAMETHYLMELAMINE ———
[HMM, HXM]

POSSIBLE SIDE EFFECTS	SIGNS AND SYMPTOMS
Nausea and vomiting	
Appetite, decreased (anorexia)	
Infection, fewer white blood cells (leukopenia)	Sore throat, cough, stuffy nose; burning when you urinate; shaking chills; diarrhea; burning (pain) when you have a bowel movement; pain, redness, swelling, and heat if you hurt your skin; temperature above 100.5°F (38°C); eyes or ears drain
Bleeding, low platelet count (thrombocytopenia)	Unexplained bruises; bleeding gums; nosebleeds; blood in your vomit may be bright red or coffee-ground-like; blood in stool may be red or black and tarry; blood in urine or sputum; headache; visual changes (loss of a portion of your field of vision or blurriness); increased flow with menses
Numbness, tingling hands and feet (peripheral neuropathies)	Clumsiness in hands and feet and/or they feel different to you, different sensation
Mood changes	Sudden mood changes; you feel "blue" or find yourself crying for no apparent reason
Hair thinning or loss (alopecia)	Hair on your head and body thins and falls out

Skin rash, itching,
  peeling, hives
  (dermatitis)
Abdominal cramps
  and pain
Diarrhea
Central nervous   Tiredness; somnolence; confusion
  system toxicity

———— HYDROXYUREA (Hydrea) ————

POSSIBLE SIDE EFFECTS

SIGNS AND SYMPTOMS

Infection, fewer
  white blood cells
  (leukopenia)

Sore throat, cough, stuffy nose; burning when you urinate; shaking chills;
  diarrhea; burning (pain) when you
  have a bowel movement; pain, redness, swelling, and heat if you hurt
  your skin; temperature above 100.5°F
  (38°C); eyes or ears drain

Bleeding, low plate-
  let count (throm-
  bocytopenia)

Unexplained bruises; bleeding gums;
  nosebleeds; blood in your vomit may
  be red or black and tarry; blood in urine
  or sputum; headaches; visual changes
  (loss of a portion of your field of vision
  or blurriness); increased flow with menses

Anemia, fewer red
  blood cells

More tired than usual; dizzy when you
  change positions; lightheadedness;
  pale membranes (lining) in your
  mouth and inner eyelids; feel cold
  more often; insomnia; nervousness

Nausea and vomit-
  ing
Diarrhea
Constipation
Skin rash, itching,
  peeling, hives
  (dermatitis)

Kidney damage, kidney poisoning — Headache; puffiness at the ankles and hands; flank pain

Mouth sores (stomatitis) — Mouth, gums, and throat feel sore (raw), burning, or different; red mouth and gums

Appetite, decreased (anorexia)

——— IFOSFAMIDE (IFEX) ———

POSSIBLE SIDE EFFECTS	SIGNS AND SYMPTOMS
Infection, fewer white blood cells (leukopenia)	Sore throat, cough, stuffy nose; burning when you urinate; shaking chills; diarrhea; burning (pain) when you have a bowel movement; pain, redness, swelling, and heat if you hurt your skin; temperature above 100.5°F (38°C); eyes or ears drain
Bleeding, low platelet count (thrombocytopenia)	Unexplained bruises; bleeding gums; nosebleeds; blood in your vomit may be bright red or coffee-ground-like; blood in stool may be red or black and tarry; blood in urine or sputum; headache; visual changes (loss of a portion of your field vision or blurriness); increased flow with menses
Blood in urine (hematuria)	You need to urinate frequently, but it is difficult to urinate; urine has pink color; low back pain
Kidney damage, kidney poisoning	Headache; puffiness at the ankles and hands; flank pain
Central nervous system toxicity	Tiredness; somnolence; confusion; seeing things that are not there; depressive psychosis

| Hair thinning or loss (alopecia) | Hair in your head and body thins and falls out |
| Nausea and vomiting | |

———— L-ASPARAGINASE (Elspar) ————

POSSIBLE SIDE EFFECTS	SIGNS AND SYMPTOMS
Fever	
Liver damage, liver poisoning	Yellow skin and yellow tinge to the whites of your eyes; nausea; fatigue; pain on right side
Kidney damage, kidney poisoning	Headache; puffiness at the ankles and hands; flank pain
Bleeding, low platelet count (thrombocytopenia)	Unexplained bruises; bleeding gums; nosebleeds; blood in your vomit may be red or black and tarry; blood in urine or sputum; headache; visual changes (loss of a portion of your field of vision or blurriness); increased flow with menses
Anemia, fewer red blood cells	More tired than usual; dizzy when you change positions; lightheadedness; pale membranes (lining) in your mouth and inner eyelids; feel cold more often; insomnia; nervousness
Central nervous system toxicity	Tiredness, somnolence, confusion
Nausea and vomiting	
Appetite, decreased (anorexia)	
Mouth sores (stomatitis)	Mouth, gums and throat may feel sore (raw) burning, or different; reddened areas on mouth and on gums

——— LEUPROLIDE (Lupron) ———

POSSIBLE SIDE EFFECTS	SIGNS AND SYMPTOMS
Hot flashes	
Pain at site of tumor occurs soon after you take your initial chemotherapy	
Blood in urine (hematuria)	Difficulty in urinating; urine has pink color and sometimes has blood clots; low back pain
Sexual dysfunction, sterility	Impotence and decreased libido, menstrual irregularities, adverse effects on fetal development (if conception occurs, drug adversely impacts the reproductive system)
Nausea and vomiting	
Constipation	
Dermatitis, skin redness and peeling at injection site	

——— LOMUSTINE [CCNU] (CeeNU) ———

POSSIBLE SIDE EFFECTS	SIGNS AND SYMPTOMS
Nausea and vomiting	

Possible Side Effects, Signs, and Symptoms

Infection, fewer white blood cells (leukopenia)	Sore throat, cough, stuffy nose; burning when you urinate; shaking chills; diarrhea; burning (pain) when you have a bowel movement; pain, redness, swelling, and heat if you hurt your skin; temperature above 100.5°F (38°C); eyes or ears drain
Bleeding, low platelet count (thrombocytopenia)	Unexplained bruises; bleeding gums; nosebleeds; blood in your vomit may be bright red or coffee-ground-like; blood in stool may be red or black and tarry; blood in urine or sputum; headache; visual changes (loss of a portion of your field of vision or blurriness); increased flow with menses
Mouth sores (stomatitis)	Mouth, gums, and throat feel sore (raw), burning, or different; red mouth and gums
Hair thinning or loss (alopecia)	Hair on your head and body thins and falls out
Anemia, fewer red blood cells	More tired than usual; dizzy when you change positions; lightheadedness; pale membranes (lining) in your mouth and eyes; feel cold more often; insomnia; nervousness
Sexual dysfunction, sterility	Impotence and decreased libido, menstrual irregularities, adverse effects on fetal development (if conception occurs before drug adversely impacts the reproductive system)

———— MAYTANSINE ————

POSSIBLE SIDE EFFECTS	SIGNS AND SYMPTOMS
Nausea and vomiting	
Diarrhea	

Mouth sores (stomatitis)	Mouth, gums, and throat feel sore (raw), burning, or different; red mouth and gums
Numbness, tingling hands and feet (peripheral neuropathies)	Clumsiness in hands and feet and they feel different
Nervousness, irritability, insomnia, fatigue	
Liver damage, liver poisoning	Yellow skin and yellow tinge to the whites of your eyes; nausea; fatigue; pain on right side
Infection, fewer white blood cells (leukopenia)	Sore throat, cough, stuffy nose; burning when you urinate; shaking chills; diarrhea; burning (pain) when you have a bowel movement; pain, redness, swelling, and heat if you hurt your skin; temperature above 100.5°F (38°C); eyes or ears drain
Hair thinning or loss (alopecia)	Hair on your head and body thins and falls out
Constipation	
Anemia, fewer red blood cells	More tired than usual; dizzy when you change positions; lightheadedness; pale membranes (lining) in your mouth and inner eyelids; feel cold more often; insomnia; nervousness

———— MECHLORETHAMINE ———— HYDROCHLORIDE (Mustargen)

POSSIBLE SIDE EFFECTS	SIGNS AND SYMPTOMS
Nausea and vomiting	
Infection, fewer white blood cells (leukopenia)	Sore throat, cough, stuffy nose; burning when you urinate; shaking chills; diarrhea; burning (pain) when you have a bowel movement; pain, red-

	ness, swelling, and heat if you hurt your skin; temperature above 100.5°F (38°C); eyes or ears drain
Bleeding, low platelet count (thrombocytopenia)	Unexplained bruises; bleeding gums; nosebleeds; blood in your vomit may be bright red or coffee-ground-like; blood in stool may be red or black and tarry; blood in urine or sputum; headache; visual changes (loss of a portion of your field of vision or blurriness); increased flow with menses
Anemia, fewer red blood cells	More tired than usual; dizzy when you change positions; lightheadedness; pale membranes (lining) in your mouth and eyes; feel cold more often; insomnia; nervousness
Mouth sores (stomatitis)	Mouth, gums, and throat feel sore (raw), burning, or different; red mouth and gums
Skin burning as needle delivering chemotherapy comes out of the vein (extravasation)	Swelling, redness, warmth, and pain over skin; notify physician or nurse immediately
Sexual dysfunction, sterility	Impotence and decreased libido, menstrual irregularities, adverse effects on fetal development (if conception occurs, drug adversely impacts the reproductive system)
Skin rash, itching, peeling (dermatitis)	
Ringing sensation in your ears or hearing loss	

——— MEDROXYPROGESTERONE ———
ACETATE (Provera; Depo-Provera)

POSSIBLE SIDE EFFECTS	SIGNS AND SYMPTOMS
Weight increase with fluid retention (edema)	Puffiness (swelling of your ankles and hands) and overall weight gain
Mood changes	Sudden mood changes; you feel "blue" or find yourself crying for no apparent reason
Breast tenderness	
Thrombophlebitis (inflammation and clotting of blood in the veins)	Pain, tenderness, and/or redness in your arms or legs (calves or thighs)

——— MEGESTROL ACETATE ———
(Megace)

POSSIBLE SIDE EFFECTS	SIGNS AND SYMPTOMS
Weight increase with fluid retention (edema)	Puffiness (swelling of your ankles and hands) and overall weight gain
Weight increase with fat deposits	Fullness or roundness of face (moon face); fat deposits between your shoulder blades; increased appetite
Hair thinning or loss (alopecia)	Hair on your head and body thins and falls out
Liver damage, liver poisoning	Yellow skin and yellow tinge to the whites of your eyes; nausea; fatigue; pain on right side

——— MELPHALAN [L-PAM] (Alkeran) ———

POSSIBLE SIDE EFFECTS	SIGNS AND SYMPTOMS
Nausea and vomiting	
Infection, fewer white blood cells (leukopenia)	Sore throat, cough, stuffy nose; burning when you urinate; shaking chills; diarrhea; burning (pain) when you have a bowel movement; pain, redness, swelling, and heat if you hurt your skin; temperature above 100.5°F (38°C); eyes or ears drain
Bleeding, low platelet count (thrombocytopenia)	Unexplained bruises; bleeding gums; nosebleeds; blood in your vomit may be bright red or coffee-ground-like; blood in stool may be red or black and tarry; blood in urine or sputum; headache; visual changes (loss of a portion of your field of vision or blurriness); increased flow with menses
Anemia, fewer red blood cells	More tired than usual; dizzy when you change positions; lightheadedness; pale membranes (lining) in your mouth and inner eyelids; feel cold more often; insomnia; nervousness
Appetite, decreased (anorexia)	
Nausea and vomiting	
Mouth sores (stomatitis)	Mouth, gums, and throat feel sore (raw), burning, or different; red mouth and gums
Diarrhea	
Fever	

Skin rash, itching, peeling, hives (dermatitis)	
Liver damage, liver poisoning	Yellow skin and yellow tinge to the whites of your eyes; nausea; fatigue; pain on right side

─────── MERCAPTOPURINE [6-MP] ───────

POSSIBLE SIDE EFFECTS	SIGNS AND SYMPTOMS
Infection, fewer white blood cells (leukopenia)	Sore throat, cough, stuffy nose; burning when you urinate; shaking chills; diarrhea; burning (pain) when you have a bowel movement; pain, redness, swelling, and heat if you hurt your skin; temperature above 100.5°F (38°C); eyes or ears drain
Bleeding, low platelet count (thrombocytopenia)	Unexplained bruises; bleeding gums; nosebleeds; blood in your vomit may be red or black and tarry; blood in urine or sputum; headache, visual changes (loss of a portion of your field of vision or blurriness); increased flow with menses
Anemia, fewer red blood cells	More tired than usual; dizzy when you change positions; lightheadedness; pale membranes (lining) in your mouth and inner eyelids; feel cold more often; insomnia; nervousness
Appetite, decreased (anorexia)	
Nausea and vomiting	
Mouth sores (stomatitis)	Mouth, gums and throat feel sore (raw), burning, or different; red mouth and gums
Diarrhea	

Fever

Skin rash, itching,
peeling, hives
(dermatitis)

Liver damage, liver   Yellow skin and yellow tinge to the
poisoning   whites of your eyes; nausea; fatigue;
                        pain on right side

———— METHOTREXATE ————
[MTX] SODIUM

POSSIBLE SIDE   **SIGNS AND SYMPTOMS**
EFFECTS

Mouth sores (sto-   Mouth, gums, and throat feel sore
matitis)   (raw), burning, or different, red
                       mouth and gums

Infection, fewer   Sore throat, cough, stuffy nose; burn-
white blood cells   ing when you urinate; shaking chills;
(leukopenia)   diarrhea; burning (pain) when you
                       have a bowel movement; pain, red-
                       ness, swelling, and heat if you hurt
                       your skin; temperature above 100.5°F
                       (38°C); eyes or ears drain

Nausea and vomit-
ing

Diarrhea

Anemia, fewer red   More tired than usual; dizzy when you
blood cells   change positions; lightheadedness;
                       pale membranes (lining) in your
                       mouth and eyes; feel cold more of-
                       ten; insomnia; nervousness

Bleeding, low plate-   Unexplained bruises; bleeding gums;
let count (throm-   nosebleeds; blood in your vomit may
bocytopenia)   be bright red or coffee-ground-like;
                       blood in stool may be red or black and
                       tarry; blood in urine or sputum; head-
                       ache; visual changes (loss of a portion
                       of your field of vision or blurriness); in-
                       creased flow with menses

Liver damage, liver poisoning	Yellow skin and yellow tinge to the whites of your eyes; nausea; fatigue; pain on right side
Kidney damage, kidney poisoning	Headache; puffiness at the ankles and hands; flank pain
Increased color of skin (hyperpigmentation)	Sunburnlike rash with or without exposure to the sun
Appetite, decreased (anorexia)	
Skin rash, itching, peeling, hives (dermatitis)	
Central nervous system toxicity	Tiredness, somnolence; confusion
Light sensitivity (photophobia)	

——— MITHRAMYCIN or ——— PLICAMYCIN (Mithracin)

POSSIBLE SIDE EFFECTS	SIGNS AND SYMPTOMS
Nausea and vomiting	
Mouth sores (stomatitis)	Mouth, gums, and throat feel sore (raw), burning, or different; red mouth and gums
Kidney damage, kidney poisoning	Headache; puffiness at the ankles and hands; flank pain
Liver damage, liver poisoning	Yellow skin and yellow tinge to the whites of your eyes; nausea; fatigue; pain on right side
Mood changes	Sudden mood changes; you feel ''blue'' or find yourself crying for no apparent reason; you may experience feelings of irritability and/or lethargy; insomnia; nervousness

Possible Side Effects, Signs, and Symptoms

Headache

Diarrhea

Appetite, de-
creased (ano-
rexia)

Bleeding, low plate-let count (throm-bocytopenia)	Unexplained bruises; bleeding gums; nosebleeds; blood in your vomit may be bright red or coffee-ground-like; blood in stool may be red or black and tarry; blood in urine or sputum; headache; visual changes (loss of a portion of your field of vision or blurriness); increased flow with menses
Infection, fewer white blood cells (leukopenia)	Sore throat, cough, stuffy nose; burning when you urinate; shaking chills; diarrhea; burning (pain) when you have a bowel movement; pain, redness, swelling, and heat if you hurt your skin; temperature above 100.5°F (38°C); eyes or ears drain

NOTE: Side effects needing immediate attention and which may occur 1 to 2 hours after the chemotherapy injection is started and continue for 12 to 24 hours; Nausea and vomiting; drowsiness; fever; headache; depression; pain, redness, and swelling at site of injection; unusual tiredness or weakness.

——— MITOMYCIN (Mutamycin) ———

POSSIBLE SIDE EFFECTS	SIGNS AND SYMPTOMS
Nausea and vomiting	
Appetite, decreased (anorexia)	
Anemia, fewer red blood cells	More tired than usual; dizzy when you change positions; lightheadedness; pale membranes (lining) in your mouth and eyes; feel cold more often; insomnia; nervousness

— 43 —

Infection, fewer white blood cells (leukopenia)	Sore throat, cough, stuffy nose; burning when you urinate; shaking chills; diarrhea; burning (pain) when you have a bowel movement; pain, redness, swelling, and heat if you hurt your skin; temperature above 100.5°F (38°C); eyes or ears drain
Bleeding, low platelet count (thrombocytopenia)	Unexplained bruises; bleeding gums; nosebleeds; blood in your vomit may be bright red or coffee-ground-like; blood in stool may be red or black and tarry; blood in urine or sputum; headache; visual changes (loss of a portion of your field of vision or blurriness); increased flow with menses
Kidney damage, kidney poisoning	Headache, puffiness at the ankles and hands; flank pain
Skin burning as needle delivering chemotherapy comes out of the vein (extravasation)	Swelling, redness, warmth, and pain over skin, notify physician or nurse immediately
Mouth sores (stomatitis)	Mouth, gums, and throat feel sore (raw), burning, or different; red mouth and gums
Hair thinning or loss (alopecia)	Hair on your head and body thins and falls out

——— MITOXANTRONE ———
HYDROCHLORIDE (Novantrone)

POSSIBLE SIDE EFFECTS	SIGNS AND SYMPTOMS
Heart damage (cardiac toxicity)	Puffiness or swelling of your hands and ankles; shortness of breath; loss of appetite; skipped heartbeat or palpitations

Sexual dysfunction, sterility	Impotence and decreased libido, menstrual irregularities, adverse effects on fetal development (if conception occurs, drug adversely impacts the reproductive system)
Nausea and vomiting	
Hair thinning or loss (alopecia)	Hair on your head and body falls out
Mouth sores (stomatitis)	Mouth, gums, and throat feel sore (raw), burning, or different; red mouth and gums
Diarrhea	
Infection, fewer white blood cells (leukopenia)	Sore throat, cough, stuffy nose; burning when you urinate; shaking chills; diarrhea; burning (pain) when you have a bowel movement; pain, redness, swelling, and heat if you hurt your skin; temperature above 100.5°F (38°C); eyes or ears drain
Bleeding, low platelet count (thrombocytopenia)	Unexplained bruises; bleeding gums; nosebleeds; blood in your vomit may be red or black and tarry; blood in urine or sputum; headache; visual changes (loss of a portion of your field of vision or blurriness); increased flow with menses
Fever	

——— PREDNISONE ———

POSSIBLE SIDE EFFECTS	SIGNS AND SYMPTOMS
Appetite increase	
Weight increase with fluid retention (edema)	Puffiness (swelling of your ankles and hands); overall weight gain

Weight increase with fat deposits	Fullness or roundness of face (moon face); fat deposits between your shoulder blades; increased appetite
Blood pressure, elevated (hypertension)	Headache; nosebleeds; vision problems
Stomach irritation and ulcers (gastric ulcers)	Heartburn; indigestion; gnawing, burning pain in stomach area; nausea and vomiting; blood in your vomit may be bright red or coffee-ground-like in appearance
Weakening of bones (osteoporosis)	No signs or symptoms of weakening of the bones until a fracture of a bone occurs; then there will be pain, swelling, inability to hold your body weight if the fracture involves the hips or legs
Mood changes	Sudden mood changes; you may feel "blue" or find yourself crying for no apparent reason; you may experience feelings of irritability and/or lethargy; insomnia; nervousness; euphoria
Skin	Acne
Muscle pain (cramps)	Leg cramps
Sexual dysfunction, sterility	Impotence and decreased libido, menstrual irregularities, adverse effects on fetal development (if conception occurs, drug adversely impacts the reproductive system)

───── PROCARBAZINE ─────
HYDROCHLORIDE (Matulane)

POSSIBLE SIDE EFFECTS	SIGNS AND SYMPTOMS
Nausea and vomiting	

Possible Side Effects, Signs, and Symptoms

Appetite, decreased (anorexia)

Mouth sores (stomatitis)

Mouth, gums, and throat feel sore (raw), burning, or different; red mouth and gums

Diarrhea

Flulike syndrome

Muscle aches; fatigue; nausea; slight oral temperature; loss of appetite

Infection, fewer white blood cells (leukopenia)

Sore throat, cough, stuffy nose; burning when you urinate; shaking chills; diarrhea; burning (pain) when you have a bowel movement; pain, redness, swelling, and heat if you hurt your skin; temperature above 100.5°F (38°C); eyes or ears drain

Bleeding, low platelet count (thrombocytopenia)

Unexplained bruises; bleeding gums; nosebleeds; blood in your vomit may be bright red or coffee-ground-like; blood in stool may be red or black and tarry; blood in urine or sputum; headache; visual changes (loss of a portion of your field of vision or blurriness); increased flow with menses

Anemia, fewer red blood cells

More tired than usual; dizzy when you change positions; lightheadedness; pale membranes in your mouth and eyes; feel cold more often; insomnia; nervousness

Muscle pain

Sexual dysfunction, sterility

Impotence and decreased libido, menstrual irregularities, adverse effects on fetal development (if conception occurs, drug adversely impacts the reproductive system)

Intolerance to alcoholic beverages	Nausea and vomiting occur with the ingestion of alcohol (beer and wine included); treatment produces same symptoms as Antabuse, a drug recovering alcoholics take to induce vomiting if they drink alcoholic beverages
Blood pressure, elevated (hypertension)	Headache; nosebleeds, vision problems
Intolerance to foods that have a high tyramine content (foods that are aged to increase their flavor), for example, cheeses, yogurt, sour cream, raisins, bananas, avocados, soy sauce, broad bean pods, yeast extracts, meats prepared with tenderizers	
Pigmentation, increased coloring of the skin	

——— STREPTOZOCIN (Zanosar) ———

POSSIBLE SIDE EFFECTS	SIGNS AND SYMPTOMS
Kidney damage, kidney poisoning	Headache; puffiness at the ankles and hands; flank pain
Liver damage, liver poisoning	Yellow skin and yellow tinge to the whites of your eyes; nausea; fatigue; pain on right side

Nausea and vomit-
ing

Skin burning as
   needle delivering
   chemotherapy
   comes out of the
   vein (extravasa-
   tion)

Swelling, redness, warmth, and pain
   over skin; notify physician or nurse
   immediately

—————— TAMOXIFEN CITRATE ——————
(Nolvadex)

POSSIBLE SIDE
EFFECTS

SIGNS AND SYMPTOMS

Nausea and vomit-
ing

Headache

Skin rash, itching,
   peeling, (derma-
   titis)

Infection, fewer
   white blood cells
   (leukopenia)

Sore throat, cough, stuffy nose; burning when you urinate; shaking chills;
   diarrhea; burning (pain) when you
   have a bowel movement; pain, redness, swelling, and heat if you hurt
   your skin; temperature above 100.5°F
   (38°C); eyes or ears drain

Bleeding, low plate-
   let count (throm-
   bocytopenia)

Unexplained bruises; bleeding gums;
   nosebleeds; blood in your vomit may
   be bright red or coffee-ground-like;
   blood in stool may be red or black and
   tarry; blood in urine or sputum; headache; visual changes (loss of a portion
   of your field of vision or blurriness); increased flow with menses

Sexual dysfunction	Number of days of normal menstrual cycle may change; menstrual flow may change; spotting during menstrual cycle may occur; you may experience hot flashes; pregnancy is still possible
Fertility increased, but you must not use oral contraceptives	

───────── TENIPOSIDE [VM-26] ─────────

POSSIBLE SIDE EFFECTS	SIGNS AND SYMPTOMS
Infection, fewer white blood cells (leukopenia)	Sore throat, cough, stuffy nose; burning when you urinate; shaking chills; diarrhea; burning (pain) when you have a bowel movement; pain, redness, swelling, and heat if you hurt your skin; temperature above 100.5°F (38°C); eyes or ears drain
Bleeding, low platelet count (thrombocytopenia)	Unexplained bruises; bleeding gums; nosebleeds; blood in your vomit may be red or black and tarry; blood in urine or sputum; headache; visual changes (loss of a portion of your field of vision or blurriness); increased flow with menses
Nausea and vomiting	
Hair thinning or loss (alopecia)	Hair on your head and body thins and falls out
Blood pressure, low (hypotension)	Dizziness; lightheadedness when changing positions and standing

——— THIOGUANINE [6-TG] ———

POSSIBLE SIDE EFFECTS	SIGNS AND SYMPTOMS
Infection, fewer white blood cells (leukopenia)	Sore throat, cough, stuffy nose; burning when you urinate; shaking chills; diarrhea; burning (pain) when you have a bowel movement; pain, redness, swelling, and heat if you hurt your skin; temperature above 100.5°F (38°C); eyes or ears drain
Bleeding, low platelet count (thrombocytopenia)	Unexplained bruises; bleeding gums; nosebleeds; blood in your vomit may be red or black and tarry; blood in urine or sputum; headache; visual changes (loss of a portion of your field of vision or blurriness); increased flow with menses
Anemia, fewer red blood cells	More tired than usual; dizzy when you change positions; lightheadedness; pale membranes (lining) in your mouth and inner eyelids; feel cold more often; insomnia; nervousness
Nausea and vomiting	
Appetite, decreased (anorexia)	
Diarrhea	
Mouth sores (stomatitis)	Mouth, gums, and throat feel sore (raw), burning, or different; red mouth and gums
Liver damage, liver poisoning	Yellow skin and yellow tinge to the whites of your eyes; nausea; fatigue; pain on right side

───── THIO-TEPA [THIOTEPA] ─────

POSSIBLE SIDE EFFECTS	SIGNS AND SYMPTOMS
Fever	
Infection, fewer white blood cells (leukopenia)	Sore throat, cough, stuffy nose; burning when you urinate; shaking chills; diarrhea; burning (pain) when you have a bowel movement, pain, redness, swelling, and heat if you hurt your skin; temperature above 100.5°F (38°C); ears or eyes drain
Bleeding, low platelet count (thrombocytopenia)	Unexplained bruises; bleeding gums, nosebleeds; blood in your vomit may be red or black and tarry; blood in urine or sputum; headache; visual changes (loss of a portion of your field of vision or blurriness); increased flow with menses
Anemia, fewer red blood cells	More tired than usual; dizzy when you change positions; lightheadedness; pale membranes (lining) in your mouth and inner eyelids; feel cold more often; insomnia; nervousness
Nausea and vomiting	

───── VINBLASTINE SULFATE ─────
(Velban)

POSSIBLE SIDE EFFECTS	SIGNS AND SYMPTOMS
Nausea and vomiting	
Constipation	

Infection, fewer white blood cells (leukopenia)

Sore throat, cough, stuffy nose; burning when you urinate; shaking chills; diarrhea; burning (pain) when you have a bowel movement; pain, redness, swelling, and heat if you hurt your skin; temperature above 100.5°F (38°C); eyes or ears drain

Bleeding, low platelet count (thrombocytopenia)

Unexplained bruises; bleeding gums; nosebleeds; blood in your vomit may be bright red or coffee-ground-like; blood in stool may be red or black and tarry; blood in urine or sputum; headache; visual changes (loss of a portion of your field of vision or blurriness); increased flow with menses

Urinary retention, unable to urinate all the urine in the bladder

Decreased urination both in frequency and amount; bladder area is enlarged

Numbness, tingling hands and feet (peripheral neuropathies)

Clumsiness in hands and/or feet; feeling of weakness in fingers and toes

Mood changes

Sudden mood changes; you may feel "blue" or find yourself crying for no apparent reason; you may experience feelings of irritability and/or lethargy; insomnia; nervousness; euphoria

Hair thinning or loss (alopecia)

Hair on your head and body thins and falls out

Mouth sores (stomatitis)

Mouth, gums, and throat feel sore (raw), burning, or different; red mouth and gums

Pain at injection site or site of tumor occurs soon after you take your chemotherapy drugs

Sexual dysfunction, sterility	Impotence and decreased libido, menstrual irregularities, adverse effects on fetal development (if conception occurs, drug adversely impacts the reproductive system)
Skin burning as needle delivering chemotherapy comes out of the vein (extravasation)	Swelling, redness, warmth, and pain over skin; notify the physician or nurse immediately

——— VINCRISTINE SULFATE ——— (Oncovin)

POSSIBLE SIDE EFFECTS	SIGNS AND SYMPTOMS
Numbness, tingling in the hands and feet (peripheral neuropathies)	Clumsiness of hands and/or feet; feeling of weakness in fingers and toes
Constipation	
Nausea and vomiting	
Blurry or double vision	
Central nervous system toxicity	Tiredness; drowsiness; confusion
Blood pressure, low (hypotension)	Dizziness; light-headedness when changing positions and standing

Skin burning as needle delivering chemotherapy comes out of the vein (extravasation)	Swelling, redness, warmth, and pain over skin; notify the physician or nurse immediately
Mouth sores (stomatitis)	Mouth, gums, and throat feel sore (raw), burning or different; red mouth and gums

TWO

Suggestions for Managing Chemotherapy Side Effects

-------- ANEMIA --------
(Fewer Red Blood Cells)

DESCRIPTION

Anemia is the decreased production of red blood cells. Chemotherapy destroys the cancerous cells and the normal cells of your body, including the normal red cells. The red blood cells in your bone marrow divide at a rapid rate and are destroyed, which may lead to your developing anemia. If you are anemic, you may become tired more quickly than before. You may be dizzy when standing, feel light-headed, become upset easily, feel chilly, or be short of breath.

DURATION

Anemia caused by chemotherapy is temporary. Your body will replenish your red blood cells in time. However, since the life span of red blood cells is 120 days, and you'll receive a number of cycles of chemotherapy in this time period, you may need a blood transfusion. Waiting for your body to replace the red blood cells would take too long. Your chemotherapy will not be given again until your red blood cell count is within a healthy range for you.

SELF-CARE MEASURES

- Rest as much as necessary to save your energy.
- Eat green leafy vegetables, liver, and cooked red meats.
- Be sure to take your iron pills if they have been prescribed.
- Change position slowly if you experience dizziness. When you first wake up, sit on the side of the bed for a minute before standing to help decrease the dizziness.
- Prioritize your activities so you will have enough energy for important activities.

OTHER MEASURES

- A blood transfusion may be necessary.
- Frequent blood tests will be necessary to monitor your degree of anemia.

CONSULT PHYSICIAN OR NURSE IF:

- You are experiencing dizziness.
- You become noticeably more tired.

- You have chest pain.
- You get short of breath when lying down.

ALSO SEE:

- Nausea and Vomiting, pages 96 to 99.
- Appetite, Decreased (Anorexia), pages 59 to 60.

——————— APPETITE ———————

Bloating

DESCRIPTION

Bloating is an overfull feeling that occurs after eating, often after having just a few bites of food. Bloating is due to the inability of the stomach and intestines to properly digest the food you eat. It may be related to the type of food you eat. Fatty, fried, and greasy foods tend to remain in the stomach longer and may cause you to feel full. Carbonated beverages, gas-producing foods, and milk may also cause bloating.

SELF-CARE MEASURES

- Eat slowly.
- Eat frequent small meals instead of three large meals a day, and increase sweet or starchy foods and low-fat protein foods.
- Sit up or walk after meals.
- Avoid fatty, fried, and greasy foods, gas-forming vegetables (e.g., broccoli, Brussels sprouts, cabbage, cauliflower, corn, cucumbers, beans, green peppers, onions, rutabagas, sauerkraut, and turnips), carbonated beverages, chewing gum, and milk.

Decreased (Anorexia)

DESCRIPTION

The cancerous cells and some normal cells of your body that multiply quickly will be destroyed by chemotherapy. The normal cells that line your mouth, stomach, and intestines may be altered or destroyed by chemotherapy. Therefore, foods and liquids may taste different to you. You may lose all desire to eat, but it is important that you continue to eat.

DURATION

Your decreased appetite is usually temporary and is relieved when you are no longer receiving a high amount or high frequency of your chemotherapy drug. However, it may take 2 to 6 weeks after the decrease or the discontinuation of your therapy drug for your appetite to return to normal.

SELF-CARE MEASURES

- Eat small, frequent snacks (six per day) that include foods you best tolerate, even if you are not hungry.
- Eat high-protein foods, for example, milk, eggs, cheese, peanut butter, and nuts. Meat products may taste bitter. Plastic rather than metal utensils may reduce the bitter taste. If you need more salt to make meat more tasty, and you are not on a salt-restricted diet, you may be able to enjoy cured meats such as ham, bacon, sausage, and corned beef, or you may want to try marinating meats in soy sauce. Meats can even be marinated in sweet fruit juices or sweet wines and cooked with fruit over them to improve their taste.

- Eat a high-calorie diet (e.g., cream, butter, margarine, sugar, syrup, jelly) if you are not overweight. You may find the same ingredients perk up your appetite, but you need more of them. For example, if you normally use 1 teaspoon of sugar on breakfast cereal, now try 3 or 4 teaspoons. Increase your use of spices and seasonings.
- Put nonfat dry milk and pasteurized liquid eggs or egg substitutes in your cooking and baking. These ingredients are an excellent source of nutrition.
- Add nutritive value to your beverages by using light cream for all or part of milk. Add 1 to 2 small dips of ice cream to milk beverages. Add 1 to 3 tablespoons of nonfat powder milk to each glass of milk.
- Take advantage of the many convenience foods available, such as frozen dinners.
- Use high-protein, high-calorie sandwich fillings. These may include eggs, chicken, turkey, or tuna salad with mayonnaise; grated raw carrot with mayonnaise and nuts; peanut butter with bananas, bacon, or jelly; cream cheese with nuts, ham, olives, or jelly; and cold cuts.
- Dilute condensed cream soups with 1 cup of milk instead of water, and add extra nonfat dry milk or undiluted evaporated milk.
- Add raisins, nuts, or dates to muffins, rolls, and cereal. Add grated cheese to biscuits.
- Vary odors and textures (consistency) of foods from meal to meal to increase your appetite.
- Drink acidic beverages such as lemonade; they may increase your appetite.
- Serve foods attractively. Socializing increases your appetite, so eat with someone whenever possible.
- Chop and serve with gravy or broth any meat or dry food that might be difficult to swallow. Try salad

dressings or mayonnaise on vegetables or meat to increase the ease of swallowing.

- Look for recipes that seem appealing. Some recipes are included in Chapter Three for your convenience. Also included is a list of foods high in protein and calories.
- Seeing food can decrease your appetite. Whenever possible, keep food out of sight except when eating. For example, use non-see-through containers; keep food in cupboards, not on the counter.
- Take supplemental vitamins if they have been prescribed.
- Clean your mouth after each meal.
- Half an hour before your meals, exercise for 10 to 15 minutes.
- Plan your daily menu in advance so that you will have many portions of food ready to serve when you do not feel like cooking.
- Have someone else prepare your meals if odors bother you.
- Perform progressive muscle relaxation or another stress reduction technique before meals. (From toe to head systematically contract and relax your muscles.) These techniques may assist in reducing tension before eating.
- Try to eat one third of your daily protein and calorie requirement at breakfast if you can tolerate breakfast relatively well.
- Eat when you are hungry even if it is not your regular mealtime.
- Limit your fluids with food. Leave room for the solid food.
- Keep easy-to-prepare snacks on hand, such as peanut butter, cheese and crackers.

CONSULT PHYSICIAN OR NURSE IF:

- You notice a major change in appetite.
- You are losing weight rapidly, for example, 5 pounds in a week.

ALSO SEE:

- Mouth Problems, Stomatitis, pages 91 to 94.
- Nausea and Vomiting, pages 96 to 99.
- Anemia, pages 56 to 58.
- Constipation, pages 71 to 72.

———— BLEEDING (Thrombocytopenia) ————

DESCRIPTION

Chemotherapy destroys the cancer cells and the normal cells of your body. It particularly destroys those cells that grow at a fast rate. The platelet cells in your bone marrow divide quickly and may be destroyed by chemotherapy. Platelet cells are necessary for normal clot formation (to help you stop bleeding). When your platelet count is low, you will have a tendency to bleed longer than you normally would. The nurse or physician will tell you if your platelet count is low, in which case you must be more careful in your everyday activities so as not to injure yourself.

DURATION

Decreased platelet cell count is temporary. Your bone marrow will replenish your platelet cells usually within

2 weeks. Your chemotherapy will not be given again until your platelet count is within a healthy range for you.

SELF-CARE MEASURES

If you have been informed that your platelet count is low:

- Watch for unexplained bruises (especially on your legs and feet). If an arm or leg is involved, elevate it above the level of the heart.
- Be careful not to bump or cut yourself. If you bleed, apply pressure over the area for 5 to 10 minutes with a bandage or clean piece of linen. Also apply ice wrapped in a plastic bag over the area once the initial bleeding has stopped.
- Avoid strenuous activity, lifting heavy objects, and bending over from the waist.
- Brush your teeth gently with a soft brush. If bleeding occurs when you floss your teeth, stop flossing for a few days, then try gently flossing again. If bleeding occurs, again stop flossing and wait another few days before trying again. Check with your physician before having dental work done.
- Do not take any type of injection unless absolutely necessary. Be sure the nurse or physician giving you an injection knows that your platelet count is low.
- If you must have blood drawn or be given an intravenous injection, put pressure on the needle site for at least 5 minutes to control bleeding after the needle is removed.
- Tell the person drawing your blood not to use a tourniquet.
- Do not use aspirin or products that contain aspirin. Check the labels of all drugs you are taking for sali-

cylic acid. If you are not sure about a drug, ask your physician, nurse, or druggist whether you should use the drug while your platelet count is low. Use acetaminophen in place of aspirin.

- Avoid blowing your nose too hard, coughing too harshly, or straining too much with a bowel movement.
- Take prescribed steroid medications with milk, food, or an antacid (e.g., Maalox).
- Avoid drinking alcoholic beverages, including beer and wine.
- Avoid tampon use during menses.
- Eat protein-rich foods and beverages.
- Drink 8 to 10 8-ounce glasses of fluid a day to keep the intestinal lining in good condition and to avoid constipation.
- Use adequate lubrication and avoid vigorous thrusting during intercourse.
- Avoid raw and coarse raw vegetables.

OTHER MEASURES

- A platelet transfusion may be necessary if your platelet count is very low and you are having bleeding problems.
- Frequent blood tests will be necessary to monitor your platelet count.

CONSULT PHYSICIAN OR NURSE IF:

- You notice any changes in your vision.
- You notice blood in your vomit, stools (which may be red or black and tarry), urine, or sputum.
- You are coughing, vomiting, or you tend to be constipated. Your physician will prescribe drugs for

these conditions. A cough syrup is usually prescribed for coughing.

- Bleeding continues after having applied pressure for 10 to 15 minutes.
- If you have a major injury or are hemorrhaging spontaneously, go immediately to the nearest hospital emergency room. Be sure to explain your chemotherapy and low platelet count.

ALSO SEE:

- Constipation, pages 71 to 72.
- Nausea and Vomiting, pages 96 to 99.

———— BLOOD IN URINE (Hematuria) ————

DESCRIPTION

Chemotherapy can be very irritating to the bladder. After the drug has been broken down (metabolized) in your body, it is eliminated through the kidneys to the bladder. High concentrations of your medicine then collect in the bladder, which is a reservoir for urine until you urinate (void). The drug may irritate the walls of the bladder, causing them to bleed. If this happens, you will pass bloody (pink with clots) urine when you urinate. Other signs and symptoms of irritation include difficulty urinating, higher frequency of urination, and low back pain.

DURATION

Chemotherapy can cause slight to severe bleeding from the bladder. This toxic (damaging) effect—in its severest form—is very rare and usually occurs only after the

— *65* —

drug has been given for many years (4 to 10 years). If bladder bleeding occurs, chemotherapy is discontinued and another drug is prescribed to treat your disease. Once the original drug that caused the bladder to bleed is discontinued, the bleeding usually subsides after several days.

SELF-CARE MEASURES

- Drink at least 2 quarts of fluid a day to flush your bladder.
- Empty your bladder as soon as you feel the urge to urinate and also before going to bed at night.

OTHER MEASURES

- A diagnostic test (cystoscopy) may be indicated to evaluate the damage to the bladder in the severest forms of this toxic effect.

CONSULT PHYSICIAN OR NURSE IF:

- You experience any of the signs or symptoms of bladder irritations: bloody urine, difficulty or burning when urinating, high frequency of urinating, or low back pain.

——————— BLOOD PRESSURE ———————
Decreased (Hypotension)

DESCRIPTION

Chemotherapy may cause your blood pressure to fall (decrease). The symptoms of low blood pressure are dizziness and lightheadedness when changing position or standing.

DURATION

Your lowered blood pressure may be a problem as long as you are receiving chemotherapy. If the amount or frequency of the drug is reduced, your blood pressure will increase. When the chemotherapy regimen is completed, your blood pressure should return to the range normal for you before you took the drug.

SELF-CARE MEASURES

- Take your time when changing your position, for example, from lying to sitting, or from sitting to standing.
- If dizziness or lightheadedness occurs, sit or lie down. These sensations will pass.

OTHER MEASURES

- Blood pressure should be checked frequently by the nurse or physician.

CONSULT PHYSICIAN OR NURSE IF:

- You experience dizziness or lightheadedness.

Elevated (Hypertension)

DESCRIPTION

Chemotherapy may cause your blood pressure to rise (be elevated). The symptoms of high blood pressure are headaches, nosebleeds, or vision problems.

DURATION

Your elevated blood pressure may be a problem as long as you are receiving chemotherapy. If the amount or frequency of the drug is reduced, your blood pressure may decrease. When the chemotherapy regimen is completed, your blood pressure will return to the range normal for you before you took the drug.

SELF-CARE MEASURES

- Take regularly the medicine prescribed to control your blood pressure. Even though you may feel good, you still need to take your blood pressure pill.
- Use measures you have found in the past that help you to relax. They may be useful in lowering your blood pressure. For example, take naps and do mild exercise, deep rhythmic breathing, yoga, or meditation.

OTHER MEASURES

- Blood pressure should be checked frequently by the nurse or physician.

CONSULT PHYSICIAN OR NURSE IF:

- You experience headaches, nosebleeds, or vision problems.

——— BONE WEAKENING ———
(Osteoporosis)

DESCRIPTION

After you have taken your chemotherapy drug for a time (up to a year), your bones may become brittle and fragile. The medicine has reduced the amount of calcium in your bones that is needed for bone strength.

DURATION

If you show signs of weakening of the bones, your chemotherapy may be decreased in amount or discontinued. It will take several months to years to reestablish the strength of the bones.

SELF-CARE MEASURES

- Walk with support if necessary.
- Avoid sudden movement (twisting, jerking).
- Avoid heavy lifting.
- Prevent falls by making your environment safe (e.g., remove scatter rugs, provide adequate lighting, install handrails).
- Take a shower rather than a tub bath. Install a handrail beside the toilet bowl.
- Take calcium carbonate (1500 mg to 2000 mg) every morning.
- Do not abruptly stop taking your medicine.

OTHER MEASURES

- Routine X-rays will be taken to monitor any weakening (decalcification) of your bones.
- Blood tests for calcium will be done.

CONSULT PHYSICIAN OR NURSE IF:

- You had a fall.
- You have pain in a bone without having fallen or otherwise injured yourself.

——— CENTRAL NERVOUS ———
SYSTEM DAMAGE (CNS Toxicity)

DESCRIPTION

Chemotherapy interferes with certain functions of your central nervous system (brain). The symptoms that may occur include tiredness, somnolence (urge to sleep), mental confusion, and depression.

DURATION

The symptoms of CNS toxicity are reversible once your chemotherapy drug is lowered in dosage or discontinued. Another drug may be prescribed as a replacement.

SELF-CARE MEASURES

- Tell a family member or neighbor if you are experiencing confusion and have him phone the physician's office and report this symptom. (With CNS toxicity a nap will not decrease the tiredness or somnolence nor will past self-care measures relieve the depression.)

CONSULT PHYSICIAN OR NURSE IF:

- You develop any of the symptoms, especially mental confusion and depression.

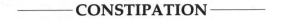

CONSTIPATION

DESCRIPTION

Chemotherapy may diminish the nerve impulses to your intestines. These impulses are needed to move the food you eat through your intestines. Once the food you have eaten has been broken down by digestion, the waste material (stool) may not move through the intestines as well as it did before your chemotherapy.

DURATION

Constipation caused by chemotherapy is temporary and is relieved when you have completed the therapy. Within a week after the drug has been discontinued, your normal bowel habits should return.

SELF-CARE MEASURES

- Eat high-fiber foods that include whole-grain cereal, bran, raw fruits, dates, prunes, vegetables, nuts, dried fruits, and raisins. Add bran to your diet, starting with 2 teaspoons per day. Increase this amount gradually to 4 to 6 teaspoons; too rapid an increase can cause diarrhea. If you have trouble chewing raw fruits and vegetables, try grating them.
- Avoid cheese products and refined grain products.
- Eat fruits like oranges, peaches, pears, and prunes.
- Drink plenty of fluids (e.g., 8 to 10 glasses a day).
- Exercise if you are able to and walk as much as you can. If you are confined to bed, do bed exercise by contracting and relaxing different muscles.
- Take stool softeners and laxatives, if approved by your physician or nurse. If you require pain medi-

cine—especially narcotics—take bulk-forming laxatives (e.g., Metamucil). Some laxatives when used continually can irritate the bowel, often making it difficult to regain normal bowel habits once chemotherapy or pain medicines are discontinued. Colace is an example of a stool softener.

- Take enemas and suppositories if stool softeners and laxatives are not effective.
- Respond immediately to the urge to defecate.

CONSULT PHYSICIAN OR NURSE IF:

- You have had no bowel movements for 3 or more days, for example, if your normal pattern is daily bowel movements and on the fourth day your bowels have not moved; or if your normal pattern is every 2 to 3 days and on the sixth day your bowels have not moved.

ALSO SEE:

- Nausea and Vomiting, pages 96 to 99.
- Numbness (Peripheral Neuropathies), pages 101 to 102.
- Appetite, Decreased (Anorexia), pages 59 to 60.

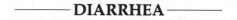 DIARRHEA

DESCRIPTION

Chemotherapy destroys the cancerous cells and the normal cells of your body, especially those normal cells that are produced at a rapid rate. The cells lining your mouth, stomach, and intestines divide at a rapid rate. As they are destroyed, you may develop diarrhea. The severity of diarrhea varies in individuals. The number of your bowel movements may increase and the stool consistency may range from very soft to liquid.

DURATION

Diarrhea caused by chemotherapy is temporary. The cell lining in your mouth, stomach, and intestines will regenerate. The diarrhea will usually stop if your drug dose is decreased or if the drug is withheld for several days.

SELF-CARE MEASURES

- Take nonprescription medicine (e.g., Kaopectate or Pepto-Bismol) to control the diarrhea.
- Drink plenty of fluid (8 to 10 glasses daily) that is at room temperature. Drinking more fluid will not cause more diarrhea, as some people may think. You need the extra fluid to replace what you have lost. Avoid hot or cold fluids since they will increase intestinal contractions.
- Take a liquid diet if the diarrhea becomes severe. Mild liquids such as fruit ades (e.g., Kool-Aid, Gatorade), ginger ale, and peach or apricot nectar are usually tolerated well.
- Avoid food that contains fat.
- Avoid food that contains roughage and bulk. Do not eat bran, whole-grain cereals, skins and seeds, beans and legumes, dried fruits, nuts, and raw fruits (e.g., dates, figs, prunes, cherries, and apples) and vegetables (e.g., lettuce, cabbage, celery, Brussels sprouts).
- Avoid drinking beverages while eating food. Avoid things that can cause gas or cramps such as beer, beans, cabbage, chewing gum, highly spiced foods,

too many sweets, skipping meals, and swallowing air while talking or chewing. Also avoid greasy foods. Allow carbonated beverages to lose their fizz before drinking them. Avoid caffeinated beverages (e.g., coffee, tea, and cola drinks).

- Eat foods high in potassium (e.g., bananas, apricots without the skin, baked potatoes without the skin, broccoli, halibut, asparagus, saltwater fish, and mushrooms). Drink peach nectar or nonfat milk.
- Eat foods high in calories and protein (e.g., fish, poultry, and ground beef that is baked, broiled, or roasted until tender).
- The severity of the diarrhea may be decreased if you drink boiled milk and eat cottage cheese, low-fat cheese, yogurt, applesauce, nutmeg in capsules or on applesauce, rice, and bananas instead of your regular meals. Nutmeg decreases the motility of your gastrointestinal tract. However, strong spices and herbs stimulate the tract and are to be avoided. When the diarrhea diminishes, gradually add your regular diet to these foods. If you cannot tolerate milk, do not drink it.*

*Milk intolerance is caused by a deficiency in lactase, an enzyme that breaks down milk sugar (lactose) in the intestine. Because the milk sugar cannot be digested properly, you may have bloating, cramping, or diarrhea. Avoid milk and milk products, such as ice cream, cottage cheese, and cheese. Try buttermilk and yogurt since the lactose in them has been changed in processing. Drink lactose-free milk substitutes (e.g., Mocha-Mix, Dairy Rich, and other soy-milk products). Some lactose-free substitutes for other milk products are also available, such as IMO, an imitation sour cream, and Cool Whip or Party-Whip, nondairy whipped toppings. Lactaid milk, available at many stores, is a product specifically designed for individuals with lactose intolerance. Toll-free hotline: 800-257-8650.

- Keep track of the number of bowel movements you have in a day to assess possible dehydration. The signs and symptoms of dehydration are dryness of skin and mouth, decreased urine volume, and sunken eyes.
- Apply nonprescription ointment that contains lidocaine if your anus is sore. A layer of Desitin or A and D Ointment, for example, applied around the anal area, can soothe irritation. Clean the area with warm water very gently but thoroughly after each bowel movement, and then pat the area dry before applying the soothing lotions.
- Keep the anal area clean by washing with mild soap and water or take sitz baths. A and D Ointment may provide soothing relief and promote healing of the irritated area.
- Avoid tobacco products.

CONSULT PHYSICIAN OR NURSE IF:

- Your diarrhea becomes severe (more than five liquid stools in a day) and the nonprescription drugs are not effective.

ALSO SEE:

- Nausea and Vomiting, pages 96 to 99.
- Appetite, Decreased (Anorexia), pages 59 to 60.

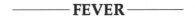 FEVER

DESCRIPTION

Fever, often accompanied by chills, can be caused by chemotherapy and is a reaction of your body to the drugs. Usually several hours after you have taken the chemotherapy drug, your temperature will begin to rise. On the days you are not receiving chemotherapy, you should not have a fever. It is important that you are aware of this pattern, because you could have a fever from an infection on days when you are not receiving chemotherapy or while you are on chemotherapy.

DURATION

Fever caused by a chemotherapy drug will continue as long as you are taking the medicine. With time, the fever will be less high even if you are still on chemotherapy.

SELF-CARE MEASURES

- Check your temperature every 4 hours while you are awake. If you do not have a thermometer, buy one and ask the nurse to show you how to read it.
- Drink plenty of fluids, for example, 2 to 3 quarts a day of ice tea, fruit ades, fruit juices, water; eat ice cream, Jell-O, and watermelon.
- Take an aspirin substitute (e.g., Tylenol) to help you feel more comfortable. Check bottle for the ingredient acetaminophen. In chemotherapy, aspirin is generally not given to lower your temperature since it could cause bleeding if your blood count is low.
- Tepid (lukewarm) sponge baths reduce fever and promote comfort.

CONSULT PHYSICIAN OR NURSE IF:

- Your oral temperature goes above 101.5°F (38.6°C) and taking an aspirin substitute has not reduced the fever.

ALSO SEE:

- Appetite, Decreased (Anorexia), pages 59 to 60.
- Infection (Leukopenia), pages 83 to 85.

———— FLULIKE SYNDROME ————

DESCRIPTION

Flulike syndrome caused by chemotherapy is a reaction of your body to the drug(s). On the days you are not receiving chemotherapy, you will not experience the flulike syndrome. It is important that you are aware of this pattern, because the flu symptoms from a viral infection that you may have will be present on days you are not receiving chemotherapy. The symptoms of the flulike syndrome include muscle aches, fatigue, nausea, slight fever, and loss of appetite. You will be getting chemotherapy even if you have these symptoms as long as the side effects are not severe.

DURATION

Flulike syndrome caused by chemotherapy usually subsides within 1 to 7 days after chemotherapy is completed.

SELF-CARE MEASURES

- Take the medicines you usually take to relieve the symptoms of the flu. Use an aspirin substitute (e.g., Tylenol). Aspirin is generally not recommended since it could cause bleeding if your blood count is low.

- Rest in bed and drink plenty of fluids (2 to 3 quarts of fluid a day).
- Gargle with warm salt water to relieve soreness in your throat.

CONSULT PHYSICIAN OR NURSE IF:

- Your symptoms become severe.
- Your temperature is above 101.5°F (38.6°C).

ALSO SEE:

- Nausea and Vomiting, pages 96 to 99.
- Appetite, Decreased (Anorexia), pages 59 to 60.
- Fever, pages 75 to 77.
- Anemia, pages 56 to 58.

———— HAIR ————

Increased (Hirsutism)

DESCRIPTION

Body and facial hair may increase. It does not mean that anything is wrong.

DURATION

The intensity of this side effect of chemotherapy diminishes as the amount of the drug is decreased. Your hair distribution will return to normal after the medicine is discontinued.

SELF-CARE MEASURES

- Tweeze or shave excess hair with electric razor. Do not use electrolysis.

- Talk to the nurse or your physician about any feelings or questions you have about your altered appearance. Do not abruptly stop taking your medicine.

CONSULT PHYSICIAN OR NURSE IF:

- Your symptoms distress you.

ALSO SEE:

- Weight, Increase with Fat Deposits, pages 124 to 125.
- Weight, Increase with Fluid Retention (Edema), pages 125 to 127.

Thinning or Loss (Alopecia)

DESCRIPTION

Chemotherapy destroys the cancerous and the normal cells of your body, especially those normal cells that are produced at a rapid rate. The hair follicle cells divide at a rapid rate and are therefore destroyed, causing some or all of your hair (scalp, eyebrows, eyelashes, facial and pubic hair) to fall out.

DURATION

Your hair will start to grow again in 3 to 4 months even if you are still receiving chemotherapy. The nature and color of your new growth of hair may be different from your pretreatment hair. If you had curly hair, you may regrow straight hair. If you had thick hair, you may regrow fine hair.

SELF-CARE MEASURES

- Keep your hair clean and wash it gently with a pH-balanced shampoo (e.g., Redken, Nexxus).
- Cut hair to shorter length if possible.
- Use a soft-bristle brush to remove tangles.
- Avoid bleaching, teasing, curlers, permanents, and hair spray; these make the hair brittle, causing it to fall out faster during chemotherapy.
- Buy wigs, scarves, and false eyelashes if you wish; they are tax-deductible medical expenses and may be covered by your insurance.
- Talk to the nurse or your physician about any feelings or questions you have about your altered appearance.

OTHER MEASURES

- The physician may place a tight tourniquet around your scalp and neck during the administration of your intravenous chemotherapy. The measure is effective with certain types of chemotherapy in causing less hair to fall out.
- The physician may place ice packs on your scalp during the administration of your intravenous chemotherapy. The measure is effective in causing less hair loss for individuals getting certain types of chemotherapy.

CONSULT PHYSICIAN OR NURSE IF:

- Your symptoms distress you.

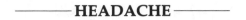

——— HEADACHE ———

DESCRIPTION

Chemotherapy may cause you to have headaches. This nervous system symptom occurs because your chemotherapy is slightly irritating to nerve tissue.

DURATION

Your headaches may occur most frequently just after you have received your chemotherapy. When the treatment is completed and the drug is discontinued, this symptom will subside.

SELF-CARE MEASURES

- Take analgesics (pain pills) as you have in the past when you had a headache. Do not take aspirin products (salicylates) if your platelet cell count is low. If you have any questions, ask your physician or nurse.
- Lying down for 1 to 2 hours after your chemotherapy may help.
- Avoid noise and bright lights if you have a headache.
- Resort to the measures you have found helpful in the past to alleviate a headache.

CONSULT PHYSICIAN OR NURSE IF:

- Your own measures do not alleviate your headache.

———HEART DAMAGE———
(Cardiac Toxicity)

DESCRIPTION

Certain chemotherapy drugs can cause changes in normal heart functioning. The drugs are particularly toxic (harmful) to the heart muscle cells. Signs and symptoms of altered heart functioning are any puffiness or swelling in your body, especially your ankles; shortness of breath; dizziness; loss of appetite; and skipped heartbeat or palpitations (fluttering) of the heart.

DURATION

The specific drug will be discontinued if any heart changes occur as a result of the chemotherapy. Another drug will be used to treat your disease.

OTHER MEASURES

- An electrocardiogram (EKG) is routinely done before the drug is given and repeated periodically (every 6 weeks) or as ordered by your physician to measure any changes in your heart function.
- The nurse or physician will listen to your heart.
- A chest X-ray will be taken.

CONSULT PHYSICIAN OR NURSE IF:

- You develop any of the signs or symptoms of altered heart function.

ALSO SEE:

* Weight, Increase with Fluid Retention (Edema), pages 125 to 127.

———— INFECTION (Leukopenia) ————

DESCRIPTION

The cancerous and the normal cells of your body that multiply rapidly will be destroyed more quickly by your chemotherapy. White blood cells in your bone marrow may be destroyed, thus making you more susceptible to infections. Even though your white cell count is low, you may not have an infection. The signs and symptoms of an infection are sore throat, cough, and nasal congestion; a burning feeling when urinating; shaking chills; burning (pain) at the anus; pain, redness, swelling, and warmth at the site of injury to the skin; and fever. You may have an infection and the injury site may not become red if you are low in a particular kind of white blood cell (neutrophil). Eye or ear drainage may be a sign of infection.

DURATION

Low white blood cell production is a temporary side effect of chemotherapy. Your body will replenish white blood cells to a healthy count usually within 4 to 10 days of treatment. You will not receive chemotherapy while your white blood count is low, but only when your white cell count is within a healthy range for you.

SELF-CARE MEASURES

- Stay away from people with colds when your white cell count is low. Stay away from crowds. Avoid going to church, shopping, movies at busy times, and so on. Your doctor will tell you if these precautions are necessary.
- Take your temperature every 4 hours while awake if you have any signs of an infection. If you do not have a thermometer, buy one and ask the nurse to show you how to use it.
- Use antiseptic mouthwashes (that contain no alcohol) daily, and have any dental problems taken care of before you begin chemotherapy to prevent possible infection.
- If you have an infection, drink 2 to 3 quarts of fluids a day. If you have a heart or kidney condition, ask the nurse or physician about this self-care measure.
- Perform excellent hygiene daily. Wash your hands before eating and after using the bathroom. After each bowel movement, clean the rectal area gently but thoroughly.
- Take rest periods during the day if you become tired.
- Always wear shoes to prevent cuts on your feet.
- Protect your hands from cuts and burns. You can wear gloves when working in the garden, wear rubber gloves when doing dishes, and use a protective pot holder or glove when cooking.
- If you do cut yourself, wash the cut promptly with soap and water and bandage it if necessary.
- Avoid getting sunburned. Wear sunscreen and avoid the sun whenever possible.
- Do not take any vaccinations unless they have been approved by your physician. Avoid contact with people who have an infection or have recently been

vaccinated against mumps, measles, polio, or small-pox (such as infants or children).

- Use a cuticle cream remover rather than picking or cutting nail cuticles.
- Use a deodorant rather than an antiperspirant, which blocks sweat glands and may promote infection.
- Women should use sanitary napkins rather than tampons to reduce risk of infection.
- Use an electric razor to avoid breaks in skin.
- Avoid rectal temperature taking and use of rectal suppositories.
- Practice deep breathing two to three times an hour, when awake.

OTHER MEASURES

- Frequent blood tests will be necessary to monitor your degree of leukopenia.

CONSULT PHYSICIAN OR NURSE IF:

- You experience any of the signs or symptoms of an infection.
- Your oral temperature goes above 101.5°F (38.6°C) or you experience shaking chills.

ALSO SEE:

- Fever, pages 75 to 77.

KIDNEY DAMAGE
(Renal Toxicity)

DESCRIPTION

Chemotherapy may cause damage to the kidneys because the breakdown products of the drug are excreted through the kidneys. The signs and symptoms of diminished kidney function are headache; change in the amount of urine; puffiness (swelling) of the body, especially the ankles; and flank pain.

DURATION

If you show the signs and symptoms of impaired kidney functioning, the drug will be discontinued and you will be given another drug to treat your disease. The headaches and puffiness of the body will subside as your kidneys repair themselves. The time it takes for repair of the kidneys varies among individuals.

SELF-CARE MEASURES

- You may be asked to increase or decrease your fluid intake.

OTHER MEASURES

- Frequent blood tests will be necessary to monitor your kidney function.

CONSULT PHYSICIAN OR NURSE IF:

- Headaches and/or puffiness of the body occur.

——— LIGHT SENSITIVITY ———
(Photophobia)

DESCRIPTION

Your eyes may be more sensitive to light or the sun while you are receiving chemotherapy.

DURATION

Your sensitivity to light will continue as long as you are receiving chemotherapy. Once the drug is discontinued, your eyes will not be any more sensitive to the light than they were before treatment.

SELF-CARE MEASURES

• Wear sunglasses to protect your eyes whenever you are in bright light.

CONSULT PHYSICIAN OR NURSE IF:

• Your sensitivity to light becomes suddenly more severe. Excessive tearing and blurred vision may also occur.

——— LIVER DAMAGE ———
(Liver Toxicity)

DESCRIPTION

Chemotherapy may cause damage to the liver. The liver metabolizes (breaks down) the drug that treats your disease. Some drugs are very toxic to the liver so the liver cannot function normally. The signs and symptoms of diminished liver functioning are a yellow tinge (color) to the skin and the whites (sclera) of your eyes, and nausea, fatigue, and pain in the right side.

DURATION

In liver damage resulting from chemotherapy, the signs and symptoms are temporary and subside within 2 weeks after the drug is discontinued. Another drug will be prescribed to treat your disease.

SELF-CARE MEASURES

• Eat small frequent snacks and meals (six per day) that include your best-tolerated foods, even if you are not hungry.
• Rest as much as necessary to save your energy.

OTHER MEASURES

• Frequent blood tests will be necessary to monitor possible liver damage.

CONSULT PHYSICIAN OR NURSE IF:

• You are experiencing any of the signs or symptoms of liver damage.

ALSO SEE:

• Appetite, Decreased (Anorexia), pages 59 to 60.
• Nausea and Vomiting, pages 96 to 99.

——— MOOD CHANGES ———

DESCRIPTION

Chemotherapy may cause you to experience sudden mood changes. You may feel "blue" or find yourself crying for no apparent reason. The contrast emotions—euphoria and hyperactivity—can be felt as well (manic behavior).

DURATION

Sudden mood changes due to your chemotherapy usually stop within 1 week after the treatment has been completed.

SELF-CARE MEASURES

- Talk to the nurse or physician and family members or friends about your feelings and moods.
- Explain to family members and friends that the mood changes for no apparent reason are due to your drug.
- Do not abruptly stop taking your medicine.

CONSULT PHYSICIAN OR NURSE IF:

- Your symptoms distress you.

—— MOUTH PROBLEMS ——
Dry Mouth

DESCRIPTION

You may experience dryness in your mouth because your saliva production has changed.

SELF-CARE MEASURES

- Good mouth care before eating will stimulate production of saliva in your mouth.
- Artificial salivas such as mineral oil may relieve feelings of dryness in the mouth.

- Drink liquids often. Drink at least 3 quarts of fluid each day. Be sure to have liquids available. Keep liquids handy at your bedside and use a humidifier during the night.
- Avoid breathing through your mouth.
- Inspect your mouth three times a day for sores.
- Suck on sugar-free hard candy or popsicles or chew sugar-free gum. These may help to stimulate saliva production. Since tooth decay is a major problem, particularly for patients receiving radiation therapy to the head and neck area, the use of sugar-free products is best.
- Suck on ice chips or ice cubes.
- Frequent cleansing of the mouth and teeth is necessary. Cleanse teeth with a soft-bristle toothbrush every 2 hours. Do not use commercial mouthwashes because they usually contain alcohol, which has a drying effect on the tissues lining the mouth. Make your own mouthwash by mixing 1 cup of warm water with 1 teaspoon each of salt and baking soda.
- Eat soft, bland foods, especially cool or cold foods with a high liquid content, such as ice cream, popsicles, puddings, watermelon, and seedless grapes. Solid foods can be made easier to swallow by adding gravies, sauces, melted butter, broths, mayonnaise, yogurt, or salad dressing. Dunking bread and other baked foods in milk, tea, or coffee will make them easier to swallow.
- If you find solid foods too difficult to swallow, you should try a pureed diet or a full liquid diet with fruit ades or nectars. Since it may be difficult for you to eat enough during this time, adding a liquid high-protein supplement to your diet will help ensure that you are getting enough protein and calories.

- Sip beverages between bites of food
- Avoid very hot, spicy, or acidic food

Stomatitis

DESCRIPTION

Chemotherapy destroys the cancerous and the normal cells of your body, especially those normal cells that are produced at a fast rate. The cells lining your mouth and throat divide quickly and may be destroyed, which leads to mouth sores. The first signs of developing mouth sores is when the mucosa (lining) appears pale and dry. Later, your mouth, gums, or throat may feel sore or different. You may be able to see reddened areas in your mouth or gums that feel raw, as if you had accidentally bitten the inside of your cheek while chewing.

DURATION

Mouth sores caused by chemotherapy are temporary and will usually be apparent 5 to 14 days after the administration of your drugs. Your body's cellular lining in the mouth and throat will grow back. The mouth sores will heal completely when the chemotherapy is completed. Chemotherapy will be temporarily discontinued if your mouth is very sore or when these sores appear.

SELF-CARE MEASURES

- Drink plenty of liquids. Keep your mouth moist. Lukewarm tea, Kool-Aid, and liquid Jell-O may be tolerated.
- Brush your teeth with a baby soft toothbrush, or

cleanse dentures after every meal to remove irritating food particles and to help prevent infection. Oral hygiene should be performed at least four times a day—within 30 minutes after each meal and at bedtime. If severe mouth sores occur, hourly oral hygiene may be necessary. Unwaxed dental floss should be used daily, but it must be used gently. If bleeding occurs when you are flossing, stop flossing for a few days and then try again. If bleeding still occurs when you floss again, stop for a few days before trying again. Bleeding can be controlled by applying pressure with a piece of gauze saturated with ice water. A water pick may be used at a low setting.

- If you wear dentures, do not use gumlike grips. If your dentures do not fit well, have them adjusted by your dentist. Do not wear dentures, retainers, or partial plates if your mouth is sore.
- Be sure to gargle with your special mouthwash if it has been prescribed (e.g., Xylocaine 2% Viscous Solution). The mouthwash contains medicine that helps ease the discomfort of mouth sores, prevents infection, and promotes healing of the sores. Gargle 15 to 20 minutes before meals to help you feel more comfortable. Some mouthwash can make you sleepy; less mouthwash is absorbed by rinsing than by swallowing. If you have esophagitis (raw throat), then swallowing is okay; if not, spit out the mouthwash. If drowsiness is a problem, you will be asked not to swallow the mouthwash.
- Avoid very hot or very cold temperatures in food as they may cause irritation.
- Make your own nonirritating mouthwash by mixing 1 teaspoon of baking soda with 1 quart of warm water. Keep this rinse in your mouth for about 1 min-

ute and repeat every 4 hours while awake. Avoid commercial mouthwashes that contain a lot of salt or alcohol (e.g., Listerine).

- Another recommended mouthwash recipe that has been helpful is 3½ ounces of Maalox and 1 ounce of viscous lidocaine plus the contents of a 25-milligram capsule of diphenhydramine hydrochloride. Shake well, use as a swish, and swallow or spit. Repeat every 4 hours as needed. Usually 1 pint with refills is prescribed. The solution should be kept in the refrigerator for an increased analgesic effect.
- Apply thin layers of K-Y Jelly or Mouth Moisturizer to your lips to keep them moist.
- Eat bland and cool, soft foods such as custards, Jell-O, yogurt, soups, and eggs. Avoid foods such as oranges, tomatoes, lemons, limes, raw vegetables, or heavily spiced foods since they may irritate your mouth more. Spicy foods that contain pepper, chili powder, or nutmeg may bother the mouth more than such spices as cinnamon, garlic, and oregano. A peeled, grated, fresh apple is easier to eat than a whole one. Hard candies or popsicles may be soothing.
- An aspirin substitute with codeine elixir can be swished and swallowed for systemic and local effects, if it has been prescribed. Systemic analgesics (pain pills) should be taken 1½ to 2 hours before meals to maximize comfort while eating.
- Look at your mouth and gums at least three times a day for any sores.
- Examine oral cavity by first removing all dental appliances. Use a good source of light. Use a glove or gauze and a tongue blade to help move the tongue and lips out of the way so you can see all surfaces. Use a dental mirror to see further back in the throat.
- If your home is heated by dry heat, a humidifier or

a steam kettle in the bedroom may help.
- Drink soft food from a cup or through a straw if you are having trouble eating with a fork or a spoon.
- Add sauces and gravies to solid foods; puree or liquefy foods if you have decreased saliva or difficulty swallowing.
- Avoid cigarettes, pipes, cigars, chewing tobacco, snuff, and alcohol.
- Ask a dentist about the daily use of fluoride gel to help prevent severe tooth decay that can develop if the flow of saliva is reduced.

OTHER MEASURES

- The physician or nurse will check your mouth frequently for sore areas.

CONSULT PHYSICIAN OR NURSE IF:

- Your mouth, gums, or throat feel sore or different, or if you observe sores in your mouth.
- Your appetite is decreased.

ALSO SEE:

- Appetite, Decreased (Anorexia), pages 59 to 60.

——— MUSCLE PAIN ———

DESCRIPTION

Chemotherapy may cause you to have generalized muscle pain.

DURATION

Your symptoms of muscle pain will continue as long as you are receiving chemotherapy. Once the treatment is completed, the pain will subside over several weeks.

SELF-CARE MEASURES

- Take analgesics (pain pills) as needed to alleviate muscle pain. Aspirin products should not be taken when your platelet count is low. If you have any questions, ask your physician or nurse.
- Use any measures you have found in the past to alleviate muscle pain, for example, a hot bath or relaxation techniques.
- Exercise with stretching motions two to three times a day if you can tolerate this activity.

CONSULT PHYSICIAN OR NURSE IF:

- Muscle pain becomes suddenly worse and is not being alleviated with over-the-counter pain pills.

———— MUSCLE WEAKNESS ————

DESCRIPTION

Chemotherapy may cause you to experience generalized muscle weakness. The reason for this occurrence is not known.

You may experience muscle twitching accompanied by feelings of thirst, drowsiness, and periods of confusion. Muscle twitching is caused by a depletion in your body of calcium, potassium, or both.

DURATION

Your symptom of muscle weakness will continue for as long as you are receiving chemotherapy. Once the treatment is completed, the weakness will subside over several weeks.

SELF-CARE MEASURES

- Rest when muscle weakness increases.
- Get up slowly on your feet.
- Prioritize your activities to be able to perform those activities important to you.

CONSULT PHYSICIAN OR NURSE IF:

- Muscle weakness becomes suddenly worse.

—— NAUSEA AND VOMITING ——

DESCRIPTION

Chemotherapy may cause nausea, episodes of vomiting, or both. The chemotherapy drugs are powerful and sometimes elicit this reaction from the body. Experiencing nausea and vomiting is not an indication of whether the drug is or is not destroying cancer cells.

DURATION

Nausea, vomiting, or both usually disappear within 1 week after you stop your daily doses of chemotherapy. If you undergo weekly chemotherapy, you are likely to experience nausea and vomiting only for 6 to 24 hours after you have received the drug. If your nausea and vomiting are severe, chemotherapy may be discontinued and another drug will be used to treat your disease.

SELF-CARE MEASURES

- Ask for an antinausea pill, suppository, or shot before each treatment, and take your pill or suppository every 4 hours on a set schedule. Antinausea (antiemetic) therapy given before nausea and vomiting are experienced is effective in more than 90 percent of patients.
- Add bananas, tomatoes, oranges, apricots, cantaloupe, dates, figs, milk, prunes, potatoes, raisins, tangerines, and unsalted tomato juice to your daily diet. These foods are high in potassium.
- Take calcium and potassium medication prescribed for you.
- Take antacid (e.g., Maalox) after taking the antinausea medicine. Avoid unnecessary movement.
- Eat small snacks (five to six times a day). Sweet or salty foods may be tolerated.
- Rest after meals. Activity can aggravate the nausea. If you recline after meals, make sure your head is 4 inches higher than your feet.
- Drink liquids frequently (but not with meals), if you are able (e.g., broth, Gatorade). It is essential that fluids with salt be given when vomiting is severe or prolonged to make up for the body's loss of water and salt. The above-listed fluids contain salt and water.
- Avoid hot foods. Their odors sometimes aggravate nausea. Try cold meat and fruit plates with cottage cheese, and small sandwiches of bland food.
- Take a pain pill, if you are in pain, before the pain becomes intolerable.

- Eat crackers or hard candy when nausea occurs; this may prevent dry heaves.
- Take fluids only for several hours after the treatment. It may be helpful to eat a light snack before the treatment.
- When feeling nauseated, try to distract yourself from the sensation by engaging in activities you particularly enjoy—for example, music, sleeping, talking about pleasant things—or try self-hypnosis or slow mouth breathing.
- Avoid greasy foods because they take longer to leave the stomach; carbohydrate-containing foods (e.g., noodles or rice) leave the stomach more quickly. The volume of food in the stomach can be reduced by avoiding liquids at mealtimes and by drinking them 1 hour before or after eating.
- Keep an estimate of the intake of fluids and output of urine to assess possible dehydration. The signs and symptoms of dehydration are dryness of the skin and mouth, decreased urine volume, and sunken eyes.
- Talk with your physician about scheduling the treatment late in the day. The effects of nausea and vomiting may cause you to lose the evening meal, but you may regain some appetite by morning. Keep track of your sickness patterns, recording the onset and duration. Most chemotherapy side effects do not last longer than 48 hours. By knowing your particular pattern of sickness you can determine better when to apply the self-care measures. Some chemotherapy drugs have a delayed onset of nausea and vomiting, for example, platinum regimens.
- Clean your mouth well before meals and brush your teeth soon after eating.
- Rinse your mouth after vomiting.

- Avoid doing your own cooking if the odor makes you feel nauseated. Sit in another room or take a walk while the food is being cooked.
- Eat slowly, so that only small amounts of food enter your stomach at a time.
- Chew your food well, so it can be digested easily.
- Do not force yourself to eat more than you can possibly manage.
- Get fresh air by sitting near an open window or outdoors.
- Cover liquids and sip through a straw if odors are nauseating.

CONSULT PHYSICIAN OR NURSE IF:

- You have been vomiting and have not been able to keep anything down for 24 hours and/or you are experiencing the signs and symptoms of dehydration.
- You are bloated, having pain or a swollen stomach before an episode of vomiting, and these symptoms are relieved by vomiting.
- Nausea persists.
- You have jerking movements of the head, neck, or limbs, that is, stiff, uneven, unintentional movements. These extrapyramidal symptoms are seen infrequently (3 percent) and result from the same antinausea drugs.

ALSO SEE:

- Appetite, Decreased (Anorexia), pages 59 to 60.

——NERVOUSNESS,——
IRRITABILITY, AND INSOMNIA

DESCRIPTION

Chemotherapy may cause you to feel nervous and irritable. You may also have trouble getting to sleep and staying asleep at night. Nightmares are not unusual.

DURATION

Your symptoms of nervousness, irritability, and insomnia will more or less continue until your treatment is completed and your drug is discontinued. If these symptoms become severe, your drug may be discontinued and another drug may be prescribed to treat your disease. Once the drug has been discontinued, you will return to your usual temperament and sleeping patterns in 1 to 2 weeks.

SELF-CARE MEASURES

- Perform any calming measures you have found in the past to relax. Examples might be taking a hot bath or removing yourself from annoying situations.
- Perform any measures you have found in the past to help you sleep, for example, drinking warm milk at bedtime and listening to soothing music at the bedside.
- Decrease intake of caffeine-containing beverages (e.g., coffee, tea, colas, cocoa).

CONSULT PHYSICIAN OR NURSE IF:

- Your symptoms are distressing you and the measures you have tried are not alleviating the symptoms.

ALSO SEE:

* Mood Changes, pages 88 to 89.

——— NUMBNESS ———
(Peripheral Neuropathies)

DESCRIPTION

Chemotherapy may affect your nervous system. You may experience numbness, tingling, or decreased sensation in your hands, feet, or both. You may find yourself suddenly being very clumsy with your feet, hands, or both. For example, opening jars, squeezing toothpaste tubes, or buttoning clothes may be more difficult.

DURATION

If your nervous system is affected by the chemotherapy, your medicine will be decreased in amount or discontinued and another medicine will be prescribed to treat your disease. The tingling or numbing sensations in your hands and feet usually disappear in time. The clumsiness also usually subsides. However, there are situations where the sensations or the clumsiness are not resolved.

SELF-CARE MEASURES

* Take care to prevent injuries to numb hands or feet (e.g., cuts or burns).
* Exercise the limb by alternately flexing and stretching its muscles four times a day for a few minutes. If you are able, short walks will satisfactorily exercise the legs and feet.

CONSULT PHYSICIAN OR NURSE IF:

- You develop any of the signs or symptoms of nervous system involvement.
- You lose feeling in your hands or feet.

——— PAIN ———

Abdominal

DESCRIPTION

Chemotherapy may cause abdominal pain. Why it occurs is not known. The intensity of the pain is related to the amount of chemotherapy you receive. Usually it is most intense shortly after intravenous administration of the medicine. Any other abdominal pain you may experience may occur for different reasons, and will not be closely associated with the pattern of drug administration.

DURATION

The symptom of abdominal pain subsides shortly after chemotherapy is completed.

SELF-CARE MEASURES

- Take pain medicine (analgesic) about 30 minutes before you know the pain to be at its worst during administration of your chemotherapy. Do not take aspirin or aspirin products if your platelet count is low.
- Do mental relaxation and stress reduction exercises: These can be learned through courses offered in

community agencies, hospitals, and through your physician or nurse.
- Change position while lying down.

CONSULT PHYSICIAN OR NURSE IF:

- The abdominal pain is not relieved with the pain medicine.
- You are in sudden and severe abdominal pain unlike the pain you experienced from your chemotherapy.

Injection Site or Tumor Site

DESCRIPTION

If chemotherapy is administered to you intravenously, you may have some pain where it is being injected or at the site of your tumor. The chemotherapy drugs are very powerful and tend to irritate the vein used for injection of your medicine.

DURATION

The pain at your injection site and at the tumor site subsides when your treatment is completed.

SELF-CARE MEASURES

- Take pain medicine (analgesics) just before your chemotherapy treatment if pain always or frequently occurs during administration of the drug. Do not take aspirin or aspirin products if your platelet count is low. If you have any questions, ask your physician or nurse.

- Ask your nurse to slow down the rate of administration of the drug.

CONSULT PHYSICIAN OR NURSE IF:

- The pain at either site (injection or tumor) continues after treatment is completed.

ALSO SEE:

- Skin Problems, Burning, pages 114 to 116.

--------- PIGMENTATION ---------

Increased Coloring of the Skin
(Hyperpigmentation)

DESCRIPTION

Chemotherapy may cause the color of your skin to darken. The two body areas especially affected are the hands and the arms.

DURATION

The darkening of your skin is permanent, although the darkening fades in some people over time (years). It does not indicate that anything is wrong, and your chemotherapy will continue.

SELF-CARE MEASURES

- Wear clothes that protect your hands and arms against the sun if you do not wish to be tanned by the sun in the areas darkened by your chemotherapy.

OTHER MEASURES

- Use sunscreen (e.g., PABA #15) for maximum protection when exposure to the sun is unavoidable.

CONSULT PHYSICIAN OR NURSE IF:

- Your symptoms distress you.

Increased Coloring of the Skin Under the Nails

DESCRIPTION

Chemotherapy may cause the color of your skin under your fingernails and toenails to darken.

DURATION

The coloration of the skin under your nails is permanent, although the coloration fades in some people over time (years). It does not indicate that anything is wrong, and your chemotherapy will continue.

SELF-CARE MEASURES

- Cover with nail polish.

CONSULT PHYSICIAN OR NURSE IF:

- Your symptoms distress you.

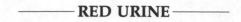

RED URINE

DESCRIPTION

Chemotherapy may cause you to have red-colored urine 1 to 2 days after receiving your medicine. It is to be expected and should not be confused with, or thought of as, blood in your urine. You will not experience any of the other signs or symptoms that occur when there is blood in the urine. As the drug is metabolized, the red breakdown product in the drug goes to the kidneys and is then excreted through the bladder when you urinate.

DURATION

As your body uses the drug, the red in your urine will disappear within 2 to 12 days.

CONSULT PHYSICIAN OR NURSE IF:

- You are not sure if your red-colored urine is the drug or blood.
- You have pain when you urinate.

ALSO SEE:

- Blood in Urine (Hematuria), pages 65 to 66.

RINGING SENSATION IN EARS (Tinnitus)

DESCRIPTION

Chemotherapy may cause you to experience a ringing sensation in your ears. Exactly how it occurs is not known, but chemotherapy somehow affects the eighth cranial nerve, which is used for hearing. In rare cases, the ringing sensation may develop into permanent loss of hearing.

DURATION

If a ringing sensation in your ears occurs from your chemotherapy, your drug will be discontinued and another drug will be prescribed to treat your disease. The ringing sensation should subside within a few days.

CONSULT PHYSICIAN OR NURSE IF:

• Ringing sensation occurs.

———— SEXUAL DYSFUNCTION ————
Feminization in Men

DESCRIPTION

Your chemotherapy may be a female hormone that inhibits the growth of your tumor. The side effects in men receiving a female hormone are breast enlargement, decreased sexual drive, and finer and sparser body hair. The occurrence and degree of these side effects is dosage-related: The greater the amount of the drug, the more increased the occurrence of the side effects.

DURATION

Feminization in men caused by chemotherapy is temporary. When your chemotherapy treatment is completed, you will return to your pretreatment breast size, sex drive, and hair texture and distribution.

SELF-CARE MEASURES

- Talk to the nurse or your physician about any feelings or questions you have about your altered appearance.

OTHER MEASURES

- Sometimes physicians recommend radiation to breasts before chemotherapy to decrease gynecomastia (enlarged breasts).

CONSULT PHYSICIAN OR NURSE IF:

- Your symptoms distress you.

Impotence

DESCRIPTION

Chemotherapy may result in your inability to gain or maintain an erection.

DURATION

Impotence may be temporary or permanent.

SELF-CARE MEASURES

- Engage in other ways of expressing affection that are satisfying to you and your partner.
- Talk to the nurse or physician about any feelings or questions you have.

CONSULT PHYSICIAN OR NURSE IF:

- Your symptoms are distressing you and the measures you have tried are not helping the symptoms.

Menstrual Irregularities

DESCRIPTION

Chemotherapy may change your menstrual cycle. You may stop menstruating or note a change in the length of your menstrual periods. Spotting between your menstruations and breast tenderness may occur. Symptoms of menopause may appear in women who stop menstruating while receiving chemotherapy.

DURATION

Menstrual irregularities will continue for the duration of your chemotherapy. Once the drug is discontinued, you should resume your normal pattern.

SELF-CARE MEASURES

- Use a well-fitting bra to relieve breast tenderness.
- Talk to the nurse or physician about any feelings or questions you have.

OTHER MEASURES

- Conception during the time of chemotherapy is a possibility. Since many anticancer drugs can damage the fetus, birth control measures should be taken.

CONSULT PHYSICIAN OR NURSE IF:

• Your symptoms distress you.

Painful Intercourse

DESCRIPTION

Chemotherapy alters the normal moisture of the mucous membranes of the penis and vagina. Decreased lubrication is particularly noticeable during sexual intercourse and may make intercourse painful for the woman.

DURATION

Decreased natural lubrication caused by your chemotherapy is temporary. Normal lubrication will return when the chemotherapy is completed.

SELF-CARE MEASURES

• Apply over-the-counter lubricants such as K-Y Jelly, Slippery Stuff, or Albane.
• Avoid products such as petroleum jelly or other ointments that have an oil base. The lubricant you use must be water-soluble.
• Change positions during intercourse (e.g., woman on top or side).

CONSULT PHYSICIAN OR NURSE IF:

• Intercourse continues to be painful.

Sterility

DESCRIPTION

Certain chemotherapy drugs decrease the number and the viability of sperm in men; women often stop ovulating. During chemotherapy many men and women become sterile but do not lose potency (ability to have sexual intercourse).

DURATION

Sterility will continue for the duration of your chemotherapy, and sperm production may be permanently impaired by the drugs. Some men regain normal sperm counts. Women may return to normal patterns of ovulation once chemotherapy is discontinued.

SELF-CARE MEASURES

- Talk to the nurse or physician about any feelings or questions you have.
- Talk to the nurse or physician about the most desirable and effective method of birth control for you, given the adverse effect of some chemotherapy drugs on fetal development.
- Talk to your partner.

OTHER MEASURES

- Ask your physician about the possibility of freezing some of your sperm for future use before you begin chemotherapy.

CONSULT PHYSICIAN OR NURSE IF:

- You are having any sexual difficulties.

───── SHORTNESS OF BREATH ─────
(Dyspnea, Pulmonary Fibrosis)

DESCRIPTION

Chemotherapy may cause permanent scarring of lung tissue and you may be short of breath. You may first notice the symptom when you are doing something that demands exertion.

DURATION

If lung tissue damage occurs in your chemotherapy, your drug will be discontinued and another drug will be prescribed for your disease. The lung tissue can regenerate itself in time (weeks) if damage from the chemotherapy has not been prolonged or severe.

SELF-CARE MEASURES

- Cut down on the number of cigarettes or cigars, or the amount of pipe tobacco, that you smoke. Best of all, stop smoking.
- Practice deep breathing at least every 4 hours while awake. Deep breathing expands the lung tissue and reduces the side effects of therapy. To deep breathe, take three deep breaths through your nose, hold your breath for 5 seconds, and then cough deeply, using your stomach (abdominal) muscles before you exhale. Coughing may not be necessary if you are not pooling secretions and you are prone to fractured bones; ask your physician or nurse.
- Rest as much as necessary to conserve your energy.
- Sit up in a chair, or rest your head in bed against several pillows, if you are having trouble breathing.
- Concentrate on soft, easy-to-chew and easy-to-

swallow foods if your shortness of breath interferes with regular meals.

OTHER MEASURES

• The physician or nurse will listen to your lungs frequently to monitor any occurrence of lung tissue damage.

CONSULT PHYSICIAN OR NURSE IF:

• You experience any increase in breathing difficulties.

─── SKIN PROBLEMS ───
Acne

DESCRIPTION

Chemotherapy may cause you to develop skin eruptions (acne) of the face.

DURATION

Acne is a temporary side effect of chemotherapy, and will disappear within 2 weeks after the treatment is completed. If you have had trouble with acne before chemotherapy, it is likely you will have acne after treatment.

SELF-CARE MEASURES

• Keep your face clean and dry. Wash your face with soap and water several times a day.
• Apply commercial over-the-counter products (e.g., Clearasil, Stridex) as directed.

- Avoid types of food that aggravated skin blemishes before you began your treatment.
- Avoid picking at blemishes.
- Do not abruptly stop taking your medicine.

CONSULT PHYSICIAN OR NURSE IF:

- Your symptoms distress you and the measures you have tried are not helping.

Burning

DESCRIPTION

Any medicine given intravenously is irritating to the vein. If the needle accidentally comes out of the vein, the surrounding area then becomes irritated. The irritation and local tissue damage is potentially more serious if the medicine is a chemotherapy drug for the treatment of cancer. Cancer drugs are especially powerful and cause severe irritation. The needle may come out of the vein for several reasons: It may not have been placed well; it may have been jarred out of the vein by movement of the body; or, after many intravenous infusions or having had blood drawn, your veins may have become brittle.

DURATION

When your physician or nurse notices the needle carrying your chemotherapy drug has come out of the vein, the medicine is immediately stopped and the needle is removed. Minor swelling and pain in the tissue should subside in several hours; more extensive tissue damage may require weeks to heal. If the burn or blister is small, the area may heal promptly. If, however, the affected area is large, you may have a non-healing sore at the injection site.

SELF-CARE MEASURES

- Apply a cold, wet cloth or an ice pack immediately to the area for 20 minutes, and then take off for 20 minutes. You can repeat this procedure for up to 18 hours.
- Apply a warm, wet cloth or a hot-water bottle after you have completed your cold, wet application.
- Apply prescription cream if it has been ordered.
- Keep the affected area clean and dry and avoid irritating the area. Wear clothes that do not cover the affected area.
- Avoid direct sunlight on the area.
- Elevate the arm on a pillow.

CONSULT PHYSICIAN OR NURSE IF:

- Needle comes out or there is burning or swelling at the site of injection.
- Your sore does not heal.

Changes in Areas Previously Treated with Radiation Therapy

DESCRIPTION

Chemotherapy may cause skin that has already been treated with radiation therapy to become red and peel or become darker.

DURATION

The skin changes may be permanent, but they do not mean that anything is wrong. Your chemotherapy will continue.

SELF-CARE MEASURES

- Apply hypoallergenic lotions to the skin area where the redness and peeling occur only if your radiation therapy is completed.
- Prevent trauma to the affected area, for example, cuts, bruises, and sunburn.

CONSULT PHYSICIAN OR NURSE IF:

- Affected area becomes cracked and infected (painful, red, swollen, warm, and with or without drainage).

Dermatitis

DESCRIPTION

Chemotherapy may cause you to develop a red, bumpy rash on your skin. The skin reaction to your chemotherapy is not unlike a rash you could get from any medicine you take. A skin rash is not an indication of whether your chemotherapy is or is not destroying cancer cells.

DURATION

There are degrees of severity of chemotherapy-related skin rashes. If you experience a severe skin reaction, your chemotherapy will be discontinued and another drug will be prescribed to treat your disease. If you have a mild skin reaction, you may continue to receive the same chemotherapy and the rash will subside when your treatment is completed.

SELF-CARE MEASURES

- Take lukewarm tub baths with ¼ cup baking soda to increase your comfort.
- Apply lotions and creams (e.g., Alpha Keri, Hydrocortisone Cream 1%, or Caladryl) that have been prescribed for you.
- Do not use soap for bathing or shampoo on your scalp if your skin is sensitive.
- Take medicine (antihistamine) prescribed for you to decrease any itching or burning.
- Avoid scratching.
- Wear cotton gloves at night if you scratch your skin while asleep.
- Avoid excessive exposure to direct sunlight.
- Use colloidal baths or oil-in-water–type lotion.

OTHER MEASURES

- A sleeping medication prescribed for you may assure a restful night.

CONSULT PHYSICIAN OR NURSE IF:

- Rash is not alleviated by prescribed drugs.

Hot Flashes

DESCRIPTION

Your chemotherapy may be an antiestrogen drug and may cause you to experience hot flashes. They occur because your drug causes the blood vessels of your skin to dilate and thus increases the flow of blood.

DURATION

Hot flashes will continue as long as you are receiving your chemotherapy. Once the treatment is completed, the hot flashes will subside over several weeks.

SELF-CARE MEASURES

- Talk to the nurse or physician about any feelings or questions you have.
- Apply cold compresses around your neck.
- Fan yourself.
- Dress in layers and discard as needed.

CONSULT PHYSICIAN OR NURSE IF:

- Your symptoms distress you.

Redness and Peeling (Sloughing)

DESCRIPTION

Chemotherapy may cause redness and peeling of the skin of your fingers.

DURATION

Your chemotherapy may be delayed, or the dosage may be reduced or discontinued if the skin on your fingers becomes red and peels. The skin will be normal again several weeks after the chemotherapy dosage is altered or discontinued.

SELF-CARE MEASURES

- Wear gloves with lanolin when you go to sleep.
- Wear gloves for protection when gardening and cooking.
- Apply moisturizing lotion frequently.
- Check for signs of infection.

CONSULT PHYSICIAN OR NURSE IF:

- You experience skin redness and peeling on your fingers, or pain.
- You think an open area is infected.

STOMACH IRRITATION AND ULCERS (Gastric Ulcers)

DESCRIPTION

Chemotherapy may be particularly irritating to the cellular lining of your stomach. In minor episodes, you may experience heartburn and a sensation of indigestion; in more extreme episodes, you may experience a gnawing, burning pain in the stomach area. If the irritated area ulcerates, you may experience nausea and vomiting. Your vomit may be bloody or coffee-ground-like in appearance (old blood). You may be bleeding in your stomach and not realize it until your bowel movements become black and tarry.

DURATION

Minor heartburn from stomach irritation does not indicate your chemotherapy should be altered. Taking an antacid drug might alleviate the symptom. If there are any indications of bleeding, however, your chemotherapy will be discontinued and another drug may be prescribed to treat your disease. The stomach ulceration will heal within several weeks after the original drug that caused the damage has been discontinued.

SELF-CARE MEASURES

- Take an antacid (e.g., Maalox, Mylanta, Gelusil, Riopan, Amphojel) to help control heartburn. Follow the directions on the bottle for taking the antacid.
- Avoid using aspirin or aspirin products, since these increase stomach irritation and bleeding. Use an aspirin substitute (e.g., Tylenol).
- Eat bland foods, for example, milk products, ice cream, custards, puddings, soft-boiled eggs, cooked cereal.
- Avoid spicy, hot (temperature), or acidic foods. Examples of acids are citrus juices and fruits, and tomatoes and tomato sauces.
- Take your medication with food.
- Avoid alcohol, caffeine, and smoking.
- If spicy or acidic foods are irritating, avoid them.
- Only stop taking your medicine if you are bleeding from your stomach (bloody vomit, bloody and tarry stools).

OTHER MEASURES

- Diagnostic tests may be ordered to examine the stomach ulcerations if there are indications of stomach bleeding.

CONSULT PHYSICIAN OR NURSE IF:

• You experience any of the signs or symptoms of stomach ulceration: gnawing, raw pain in the stomach region, bloody vomit, bloody and tarry stools.

———— SWALLOWING DIFFICULTY ————

DESCRIPTION

Difficulty in swallowing may occur because the mucous membranes (lining) of the mouth and throat are affected.

SELF-CARE MEASURES

• Chew your food well to facilitate ease of swallowing.
• Avoid lying down immediately after eating. When you are lying down, keep your head elevated.
• Choose foods with a consistent texture (such as oatmeal) instead of foods with varied textures (such as stew). They may be easier to swallow.

———— TASTE AND SMELL CHANGES ————

DESCRIPTION

Chemotherapy may cause changes in your sensations of taste and smell. Foods may taste bitter or rancid and you may develop aversions to eggs, fish, meat, poultry, fried foods, or tomatoes and tomato products. These changes occur because your drug alters the receptor cells in your mouth that send impulses to your brain telling you what flavor you are tasting or what odor you are smelling.

DURATION

Your symptoms of altered taste, smell, or both will continue as long as you are receiving chemotherapy. The changes in sensation tend to be most pronounced when you first begin treatment. Once the treatment is completed, your sensations of taste and smell should return to normal after several weeks.

SELF-CARE MEASURES

• Look for alternate foods that are palatable and are equally good sources of protein, like cottage cheese, yogurt, milk, ice cream, and peanut butter. A vegetarian or Chinese cookbook can provide useful non-meat, high-protein recipes.
• Prepare foods that look and smell appetizing. Fresh fruits, gelatin salads, and lettuce have been found to be appealing and well tolerated.
• Use seasoning—including lemon juice, mint, and basil—to help improve the taste and aroma of food. Also try extra sugar and salt. Do not try to follow any particular rule in seasoning; use your imagination and experiment. Marinating meats may help.

CONSULT PHYSICIAN OR NURSE IF:

• Your symptoms distress you and the measures you have tried are not helping.

ALSO SEE:

• Appetite, Decreased (Anorexia), pages 59 to 60.

—— URINE RETENTION ——

DESCRIPTION

Chemotherapy may prevent you from passing all the urine that is in your bladder. The signs and symptoms of this side effect are decreased urges to urinate, urinating small amounts in a dribbling stream, and a sensation of fullness in your bladder. The drug affects the nerves to the bladder and thereby decreases the impulses to the brain that initiate the "need-to-urinate" message.

DURATION

The symptom will continue as long as you are receiving chemotherapy. As with all side effects of chemotherapy, there is variation in the intensity of the experienced side effect. If you have retention of urine in its mildest form, a diuretic may be prescribed. If it does not work, your drug may be reduced in amount. If your retention of urine is marked, your drug will be discontinued and another drug will be given to treat your disease. Once the original drug has been discontinued, urinary retention will subside over weeks or months, depending on the severity of nerve involvement.

SELF-CARE MEASURES

- Drink 2 to 3 quarts of fluid a day to dilute the urine in your bladder.
- Urinate every 4 hours while awake and prior to bedtime.
- Ask the nurse or physician how to perform Credé's method (which is putting external pressure on your bladder to assist you to urinate).

OTHER MEASURES

- Your physician or nurse may insert a catheter (a plastic or rubber tube) into your bladder to monitor your retention of urine.

CONSULT PHYSICIAN OR NURSE IF:

- You are unable to urinate during a 10-hour period when you have been drinking fluids.

——— WEIGHT INCREASE ———
Fat Deposits

DESCRIPTION

Chemotherapy may increase the fatty tissue in your body. You may experience fullness or rounding of the face (moon face) and fat deposits between your shoulder blades. These fat deposits are to be expected and do not mean that anything is wrong. Chemotherapy may cause an increase in appetite, which is expected. Your medicine causes these side effects by changing the breakdown (metabolism) of the fats contained in your food.

DURATION

The intensity of these side effects (fat deposits or increase in appetite) decreases as the amount of the drug you are taking is lowered. Once the treatment is over, the fat deposits may return to normal. Your appetite will return to normal.

SELF-CARE MEASURES

- Try to stay at your normal weight, if you are not overweight. If you gain 5 pounds, eat nutritious, low-calorie foods, for example, raw vegetables, fruits, low-fat cheeses, and margarine.
- Engage in activities that divert your attention from food.
- Avoiding concentrated sweets (sugar, honey, candy) may help you stay at your normal weight and may decrease rounding of the face.

CONSULT PHYSICIAN OR NURSE IF:

- You need some guidance with your diet.

Fluid Retention (Edema)

DESCRIPTION

Chemotherapy may cause you to retain excess fluid in your body. The excess fluid will be most noticeable in swelling of the ankles or hands or in weight gain. Clothes may become too tight.

DURATION

There are degrees of fluid retention. Slight symptoms may require a diuretic (water pill) prescription. If it is not effective, it may be necessary to decrease drug dosage. With severe retention of fluids, your drug may be discontinued. Once the drug has been discontinued, the problem subsides within several days.

SELF-CARE MEASURES

- Elevate your feet as much as possible. Do not stand in one place for a long time. Do not cross your legs or wear tight-fitting clothes, girdles, or tight shoes. Continue to wear TED hose or Jobst stockings.
- Restrict the amount of salt you eat or the amount of fluid you drink if your fluid retention is severe. Your doctor will tell you if this must be done, but do not eat very salty foods (e.g., pork, ham, bacon, tomato juice, nuts, bouillon, potato chips and other snack foods, canned soups, solid cheese, salted crackers, celery salt, soy or Worcestershire sauce, catsup, canned meats, fish, corned beef, sausage, or peanut butter).
- Take your medicine (diuretic) if prescribed, and include foods high in potassium in your diet. Potassium-rich foods are apricots, bananas, cantaloupe, dates, figs, milk, orange juice, potatoes, prunes, raisins, tangerines, and unsalted tomato juice. Your doctor may also prescribe a commercial potassium supplement.
- Try salt substitutes such as Co-Salt and Adolph's Salt Substitute. Some salt substitutes taste better than others, so try several brands. Also, some substitutes contain sodium, so read the label and do not buy those that contain sodium.
- Weigh yourself daily and check your body (ankles, feet, hands, and area at base of spinal column) for edema.
- Change body position frequently (every 2 hours) to prevent skin breakdown in edematous areas.
- Do not abruptly stop taking your medicine.

CONSULT PHYSICIAN OR NURSE IF:

- You experience a sudden or severe degree of fluid retention.
- You experience shortness of breath when exerting yourself or when coughing.
- Feet or hands become cool to touch.
- You have a concurrent kidney disease before you increase your intake of potassium or try a salt substitute.

THREE

Nutrition Supplement

FOODS HIGH IN PROTEIN AND CALORIES

The following foods may be added to regular meals and used as between-meal snacks.

MILK GROUP

Milk: Whole low-fat, nonfat dry, evaporated, malted, and buttermilk; cheese; cottage cheese; cream cheese; ice cream; custards; yogurt; cream soup; eggnog; milk puddings; milkshakes; whipping cream; light cream

MEAT GROUP

Meatballs; poultry; sausage; fish; beef; lamb; tuna; veal

VEGETABLES AND FRUITS

Apricots, raisins, and other dried fruit; peas, corn, potatoes; fruit juices; beans and legumes

DESSERTS AND OTHERS

Cheesecake, cream pies; gravies; salad dressings; mayonnaise; gelatin; honey; jellies; sauces; margarine; cookies; sherbet; crackers; fruit; butter; sugar; soft drinks

BREAD AND CEREAL GROUP

Pastas; rice; bran muffins; hot and cold cereals

OTHER PROTEIN SOURCES

Eggs; nuts

———— A SAMPLE OF ———— NUTRITIONAL SUPPLEMENTS

PRODUCTS

MANUFACTURERS

Liquid Nutrition (may require doctor's prescription)

PRODUCTS	MANUFACTURERS
Citrotein (12-oz cans): Lactose-free, low-fat, high-protein supplement; artificially flavored orange or punch drink	Sandoz Nutrition Minneapolis, MN 55416
Ensure, Ensure Plus, Ensure HN, Ensure HN Plus (8-oz cans): Lactose-free, high-calorie, high-protein supplement; available in vanilla, chocolate, strawberry, eggnog, black walnut, and coffee	Ross Laboratories Columbus, OH 43216
Meritene (powder, 1-lb cans; liquid, 10-oz cans): High-calorie milk-based supplement; available in plain, eggnog, and chocolate	Sandoz Nutrition Minneapolis, MN 55416

Resource, Resource Plus (8-oz boxes): Lactose-free liquid supplement; available in vanilla, chocolate, and strawberry	Sandoz Nutrition Minneapolis, MN 55416
Carnation Instant Breakfast (7½-oz packets): Powdered supplement designed to be added to 8 ounces of milk	Carnation Los Angeles, CA 90036
Enrich (8-oz cans): High-fiber, lactose-free supplement	Ross Laboratories Columbus, OH 43216
Sustacal, Sustacal HC (8-oz cans): high-calorie, high-protein, lactose-free supplement; available in vanilla, chocolate, and strawberry	Mead Johnson Laboratories Evansville, IN 47721

Food Components (not nutritionally complete)

Polycose (powder, 14-oz cans; liquid, 4-oz bottles): High-calorie carbohydrate supplement	Ross Laboratories Columbus, OH 43216
Promod (9.7-oz cans): Powdered protein supplement	Ross Laboratories Columbus, OH 43216
Propac: Powdered protein supplement	Sherwood Medical St. Louis, MO 63103

Elemental Formulas (may require doctor's prescription)

Isotein HN: Mild vanilla-flavored partially digested formula	Sandoz Nutrition Minneapolis, MN 55416
Tolerex, Vivonex T.E.N. with flavor packets: Mild vanilla-flavored partially digested formula	Norwich Eaton Pharmaceutical, Inc. Norwich, NY 13815
Vital HN: Mild vanilla-flavored partially digested formula	Ross Laboratories Columbus, OH 43216

————— RECIPES —————

BLACK WALNUT ENSURESHAKE   *1 serving*

2 tablespoons chocolate sauce
½ cup Black Walnut Ensure
2 scoops vanilla ice cream

1. Dissolve refrigerated chocolate sauce in cold Black Walnut Ensure.
2. Pour mix into blender and blend until smooth.
3. Add ice cream and blend to desired consistency.

CHOCOLATE ENSURESHAKE   *1 serving*

¼ cup chocolate sauce
2 scoops vanilla ice cream
½ cup Vanilla Ensure

1. Add refrigerated chocolate sauce to cold Vanilla Ensure. Stir vigorously until dissolved.
2. Pour mix into blender and blend until smooth.
3. Add ice cream and blend to desired consistency.

Additional suggestions for increasing food intake are provided in the publication *Eating Hints* available from the National Cancer Society (toll-free number 1-800-4-CANCER). Nutritional programs and numerous recipes for the cancer patient can be found in E. H. Rosenbaum, C. N. Stitt, H. Drosin, and I. Rosenbaum. "Nutrition for the cancer patient." In E. H. Rosenbaum and I. R. Rosenbaum (eds.), *A Comprehensive Guide for Cancer Patients and Their Families.* Bull Publishing Co., Palo Alto, Calif., 1980.

CREAMY CARROT AND POTATO SOUP   4 servings

2 tablespoons butter or margarine
1 chopped onion
1 cup shredded carrots
3 medium peeled and diced potatoes
2 cups chicken broth or stock
1 cup light cream
2 tablespoons chopped parsley
1/3 cup grated cheddar cheese
Salt and pepper to taste

1. Melt butter or margarine in a large saucepan.
2. Add onion and cook until tinted, but do not brown.
3. Add carrots, potatoes, and season with salt and pepper.
4. Cook for 5 minutes on medium heat, stirring often.
5. Stir in chicken broth and simmer for 15 minutes or until potatoes and carrots are soft.
6. Puree in blender and return to saucepan.
7. Stir in cream and reheat but do not boil.
8. Garnish each serving with parsley and cheddar cheese.

OPTIONAL: For increased calories, add 3 teaspoons of Polycose powder or 3 teaspoons of dry milk powder.

CHOCO-COFFEE-BANANA SHAKE   1 serving

1 teaspoon instant coffee dissolved in 1 ounce of hot water
½ cup chocolate ice cream
½ banana
½ cup half-and-half

1. Put all ingredients in blender and blend until smooth.

OPTIONAL: For added calories and protein add 1 tablespoon of dry milk powder or ¼ cup of liquid egg substitute.

CINNAMON APPLE PANCAKES   6 or 7 4-inch
pancakes

1 cup all-purpose flour (sifted)
1 tablespoon baking powder
½ teaspoon salt
½ teaspoon cinnamon
1 slightly beaten medium egg
1¼ cups Vanilla Ensure
2 tablespoons salad oil
½ cup finely chopped apple
vegetable shortening

1. Sift together flour, baking powder, salt, and cinnamon.
2. Combine egg, Ensure, and oil in a small bowl.
3. Add liquid ingredients and apple to dry ingredients. Stir until moistened.

4. Fry pancakes in a small amount of vegetable shortening on a hot griddle or an electric frying pan preheated to 375°F.

If thinner pancakes are desired, pour batter onto griddle and spread with back of spoon. Leftover batter may be refrigerated for use the next day.

VANILLA ENSURE IMITATION ICE CREAM
(Refrigerator Tray Method)   1 quart

1½ teaspoons unflavored gelatin
2 tablespoons cold water
3 tablespoons sugar
2 tablespoons light corn syrup
1½ cups Vanilla Ensure
2 tablespoons and 1 teaspoon corn oil
1 teaspoon vanilla extract (if desired)

1. Soften gelatin in cold water. Add sugar and corn syrup; heat slowly to dissolve sugar and gelatin.
2. Combine Ensure, corn oil, and gelatin–sugar solution. Mix well and pour into a blender. Blender capacity should be at least 5 cups. Blend until thick and creamy.
3. Add vanilla extract, if desired, and mix well. Alternately, fruits such as strawberries, pineapple, or peaches may be added to the blender at this point. They should be well pureed and blended.
4. Pour blended mix into an ice cube tray or loaf pan and freeze until very icy.
5. Turn into blender and blend until smooth. (Stop at this point for a delicious Ensureshake!)
6. Return to freezer and freeze until firm. Allow to soften slightly before serving.

VANILLA ENSURE IMITATION ICE CREAM
(Ice Cream Machine Method) *1 quart*

1½ tablespoons unflavored gelatin
2 tablespoons cold water
3 tablespoons sugar
2 tablespoons light corn syrup
1½ cups Vanilla Ensure
2 tablespoons and 1 teaspoon corn oil
1 teaspoon vanilla extract (if desired)

1. Soften gelatin in cold water. Add sugar and corn syrup; heat slowly to dissolve sugar and gelatin.
2. Combine Ensure, corn oil, and gelatin–sugar solution. Mix well and pour into a blender. Blender capacity should be at least 5 cups. Blend until thick and creamy.
3. Add vanilla extract, if desired, and mix well. Alternately, fruits such as strawberries, pineapple, or peaches may be added to the blender at this point.
4. Pour blended mix into ice cream machine and follow manufacturer's instructions.

BLACK WALNUT ENSURE IMITATION ICE CREAM
1½ quarts

1 cup (approx. 8) marshmallows
1 cup corn syrup
¼ cup sugar
2 cups Black Walnut Ensure
1 cup whipping cream, whipped

1. Combine marshmallows, corn syrup, sugar, and ½ cup Ensure in saucepan. Heat until marshmallows melt, stirring frequently.
2. Add remaining 1½ cups Ensure. Freeze in a 9-by-5-by-3-inch pan until solid.
3. Remove from freezer and allow to stand 5 minutes at room temperature. Break up with wooden spoon.
4. Fold in whipped cream.
5. Pour mixture back into loaf pan. Cover with foil. Freeze until firm.

BUTTERSCOTCH PUDDING   4 servings

2 cups (16 oz) Vanilla Resource Liquid or Resource Plus
1 package (3⅝ oz) butterscotch pudding (can be instant)

1. Combine in saucepan.
2. Over medium heat, bring to full boil while stirring constantly. Pudding will thicken as it cools.
3. Pour into a bowl or individual serving dishes.
4. Cover with waxed paper or plastic wrap and refrigerate.

CREAMY HOT CEREAL   2 servings

1 cup water
1 cup (8 oz) Vanilla Resource Liquid or Resource Plus
1/3 cup dry cream of wheat cereal (not instant)
1 teaspoon brown sugar
1/2 teaspoon salt (optional)

1. Bring water and Resource Liquid to a boil in saucepan.
2. Slowly add dry cereal, stirring constantly.
3. Bring to a boil again, stirring constantly, and continue cooking until thick.
4. Stir in brown sugar. Salt to taste.

PART II

Radiation Therapy

WHAT IS RADIATION TREATMENT?

Radiation treatment (also called radiotherapy, or cobalt treatment, or irradiation) is the use of high-energy rays to stop cancer cells from growing and multiplying. In external radiation treatment, a machine—at some distance from you—beams high-energy rays to the spot where the cancer is in your body. This type of radiation treatment is similar to having an X-ray taken of a broken bone, but in cancer treatment the dose of radiation (measured in rads or grays) is larger and is usually given daily over 4 to 6 weeks, so that you gain maximum benefit and experience minimal side effects. You do not become radioactive during this treatment and can continue to live normally.

In internal radiation treatment, exact amounts of radioactive material (implants) are placed inside your body, usually in a body cavity like the vagina or into a tumor of the prostate or breast. The implant is left there for a few days. For internal radiation, you have to stay in the hospital for several days while the radioactive implant works on the tumor. Suggestions for managing the side effects of internal radiation therapy have not been included in this book, since the information was designed for outpatients and not those in the hospital.

High-energy rays beamed at a specific area in your body affect all rapidly growing cells only in the area being treated (cancer cells and normal cells), which is why people receiving radiation treatment may have side effects. For example, the normal cells that grow rapidly are hair follicle cells, bone marrow cells, and the cells of the mucous lining of the mouth, stomach, and intestines. The rapidly dividing normal cells that are injured are replaced by healthy cells sometimes before the radiation treatment is completed and usually once the treatment is over. If you experience a side effect with your radiation treatment, it does not mean that something is wrong or that radiation is or is not destroying tumor cells. Remember that side effects will only occur in the body site being treated with radiation therapy.

This part of the book will help you to recognize any signs or symptoms you experience during (external) radiation therapy. If you are aware of what side effects to expect, you can alert your physician or nurse when you notice them and before they become severe.

This part of the book lists suggestions for managing thirty-four side effects that may occur during or after radiation therapy treatments. Following an alphabetical listing of the body sites being treated and the possible side effects for each category are suggestions for treatment.

COMMONLY AFFECTED SITES AND SIDE EFFECTS OF RADIATION THERAPY

ABDOMEN AND PELVIS

Appetite
  Bloating
  Decreased (anorexia)
Bladder irritation (cystitis)
Diarrhea
Nausea and vomiting
Sexual dysfunction
  Impotence
  Menstrual changes
  Painful intercourse
  Sterility
Skin reactions

ARMS AND LEGS

Lhermitte's sign, decreased function
Skin reactions
Weight, increase with fluid retention (edema)

CHEST AND BREAST

Appetite
  Decreased (anorexia)
  Difficulty in swallowing (esophagitis)
  Radiation pneumonitis, difficulty in breathing
  Skin reactions

HEAD AND NECK

Difficulty in swallowing (esophagitis)
Ear inflammation (otitis media)
Eye inflammation (conjunctivitis)
Hair, thinning or loss (alopecia)
  Mouth sores (stomatitis)
  Mucositis
  Dry mouth
Skin reactions
Taste and smell changes
Tooth decay
Trismus, disturbance of chewing muscles

LARGE AREAS OF RADIATION TREATMENT AND/OR HIGH DOSAGE OF RADIATION

Bone marrow depression
Anemia, fewer red blood cells
Bleeding, decreased platelet count (thrombocytopenia)
Infection, fewer white blood cells (leukopenia)
Radiation syndrome (fatigue, malaise, anorexia, diarrhea, nausea, and vomiting)
  Skin reactions
  Weight, increase with fluid retention (edema)

FOUR

Suggestions for Managing Radiation Therapy Side Effects

———— ANEMIA ————

DESCRIPTION

Depending on the radiation amount and site, the blood-producing ability of bone marrow may become decreased. Radiation to the pelvis, bones, and chest where the bone marrow is located can cause marrow depression. Radiation affects the cancer cells and the normal cells in your body that are produced at a rapid rate. The red blood cells in your bone marrow are cells that divide rapidly, and many are injured by radiation therapy, which may lead to your developing anemia. If you are anemic, you may tire more quickly than you did before. You may also be dizzy when standing, feel light-headed, become upset easily, feel chilly, be short of breath, or have a fast pulse.

DURATION

Anemia caused by radiation treatment is temporary. Your body's bone marrow will begin to replenish the red blood cells, but this process takes time; thus, a blood transfusion is usually given. If you are still anemic, your treatment may be postponed until your red blood cell count is within a normal range for you.

SELF-CARE MEASURES

- Rest as much as necessary to save your energy.
- Change position slowly if you experience dizziness. When you first wake up, sit at the side of the bed for a minute before standing to help decrease the dizziness.
- Exercise your feet and lower legs while sitting and before standing.

CONSULT PHYSICIAN OR NURSE IF:

- You experience dizziness, chills, shortness of breath, marked tiredness, or fast pulse.

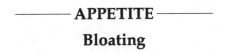

——— APPETITE ———
Bloating

DESCRIPTION

Bloating is a feeling of being overfull, often after you have eaten just a few bites. Bloating means your stomach and intestines cannot properly digest the food you eat. It may be related to the type of food you eat. Fatty, fried, and greasy food tends to remain in the stomach longer and may cause you to feel full. Carbonated beverages, gas-producing foods, and milk may also cause bloating.

SELF-CARE MEASURES

- Eat six small meals instead of three large meals a day, and increase sweet or starchy foods and low-fat protein foods.
- Chew your food very well and eat slowly.
- Sit up or walk after meals.
- Avoid consumption of fatty, fried, and greasy foods, gas-forming vegetables (e.g., broccoli, Brussels sprouts, cabbage, cauliflower, corn, cucumber, beans, green peppers, rutabagas, sauerkraut, and turnips), carbonated beverages, chewing gum, and milk.

CONSULT PHYSICIAN OR NURSE IF:

- Bloating is associated with weight gain (to rule out ascites).

Decreased (Anorexia)

DESCRIPTION

The cancer cells and the normal cells in the body site where you are receiving your radiation therapy will be injured. In radiation treatment to the chest, breast, abdomen, and pelvis some of the normal cells that line the mouth, stomach, and intestines may be changed or injured. Food and liquids may taste differently or you may lose the desire to eat. It is important that you continue to eat to help your body restore itself.

DURATION

Your appetite will only be low temporarily and will be normal again after your radiation treatment is over. It may take 2 to 6 weeks after treatment for your appetite to return to normal.

SELF-CARE MEASURES

- Eat small, frequent snacks (six per day) of the foods you best tolerate, even when you are not hungry.
- Eat high-protein foods, for example, milk, eggs, cheese, peanut butter, nuts, and legumes such as dried beans and peas. Meat products can taste bitter, but the bitter taste may be disguised or removed by pureeing meats in a blender for use in gravies and as soup stock.
- Eat a high-calorie diet (e.g., cream, butter, margarine, sugar, mayonnaise, sour cream, honey, syrup, jelly) unless you are overweight. You will need the same ingredients to perk your appetite as before, but more of them. For example, if you normally take 1 teaspoon of sugar on breakfast cereal, try 3 or 4. Increase the amount of spices, seasonings, and flavoring extracts.
- Put nonfat dry milk and pasteurized egg substitutes in your cooking and baking. These ingredients are an excellent source of protein.
- Enhance the nutritive value of beverages by adding the following: light cream or Ensure to all or part of the milk or coffee you drink; one or two small dips of ice cream to milk beverages; one package of nonfat milk to each glass of milk for drinking and cooking.
- Use high-protein, high-calorie sandwich fillings like eggs, chicken, turkey, or tuna salad with mayonnaise;

grated raw carrot with mayonnaise and nuts; peanut butter with bacon or jelly; cream cheese with nuts, ham, olives, or jelly; cold cuts and avocados.

- Dilute condensed cream soups with 1 cup of milk instead of water, and add extra nonfat dry milk or undiluted evaporated milk. Add strained and junior baby meats to soups and casseroles.
- Add raisins, nuts, or dates to muffins, rolls, and cereal. Add grated cheese to biscuits.
- Vary the odor and texture of food from meal to meal to increase your appetite. Sometimes cooking odors may seem offensive. If they are, have someone else do the cooking and avoid the cooking area before mealtime. When friends and family want to help, ask them to prepare meal-sized portions of appealing foods in freezer or refrigerator containers.
- Drink acidic beverages such as lemonade, orange juice, and tomato juice; they may increase your appetite.
- Serve foods attractively. Sometimes smaller but more frequent portions are less overwhelming. Socializing increases the appetite; eat with someone whenever possible.
- Look for recipes that seem appealing. Nutritional programs and many recipes for the cancer patient can be found in E. H. Rosenbaum, C. N. Stitt, H. Drosin, and I. Rosenbaum. "Nutrition for the Cancer Patient." In E. H. Rosenbaum and I. R. Rosenbaum (eds.), *A Comprehensive Guide for Cancer Patients and Their Families.* Bull Publishing Co., Palo Alto, Calif., 1980. Also helpful is *Eating Hints,* published by the Office of Cancer Communications, National Cancer Institute, Bethesda, Md.; toll-free number 1-800-4-CANCER.
- Looking at food can decrease your appetite. Whenever possible, keep food out of sight until you are

ready to eat. For example, use non-see-through containers; keep foods in the cupboard, not on the counter. Remove all unpleasant sensory stimuli from the environment at mealtime (e.g., the emesis basin, bedpan, and loud noises).

- Take more vitamins if they have been prescribed.
- Rinse your mouth after each meal.
- About half an hour before your meals exercise for 10 to 15 minutes, or rest if you are tired. Fatigue is usually greatest 2 to 4 hours after radiation therapy. Take this fact into consideration when planning meals. A nap before mealtime may be beneficial.
- Plan your daily menu in advance so that you will have many portions of food ready to eat when you do not feel like cooking.
- Do progressive muscle relaxation or other stress-reducing exercises before meals; these may help reduce tension before eating.
- Try to eat one third of your daily protein and calorie requirement at breakfast if you tolerate breakfast relatively well.
- Talk with your nurse or dietitian about what liquid commercial preparation high in protein and calories you should include in your meals.
- Take analgesics ½ to 1 hour before mealtime if pain is present.
- Do comparison shopping before buying nutritional supplements. Many are available in drugstores or in grocery stores. Ross Laboratories provides a home shopping service. Contact the local sales representative or your local American Cancer Society for information.
- Weigh yourself twice a week.

CONSULT PHYSICIAN OR NURSE IF:

- You notice a major change in appetite.
- You are losing weight rapidly (e.g., a loss of 2 to 3 pounds in a week). If you are overweight, do not try to lose weight until you have finished your treatments.

ALSO SEE:

- Mouth Problems, Stomatitis, pages 164 to 167.
- Nausea and Vomiting, pages 167 to 170.
- Anemia, pages 144 to 145.
- Swallowing Difficulty (Esophagitis), pages 181 to 183.

——— BLADDER IRRITATION ———
(Cystitis)

DESCRIPTION

The cells lining your bladder may be damaged by radiation to the bladder area, which can lead to bladder wall irritation. You may need to urinate frequently and may experience burning and urgency; you may experience spasmlike pain when voiding; also, you may find shreds of mucus or small amounts of blood in your urine.

DURATION

Bladder irritation caused by radiation treatment is temporary. The cell lining in the bladder will renew itself. The bladder irritation will heal when treatment is completed.

SELF-CARE MEASURES

- Drink at least 2 to 3 quarts of fluid daily to reduce the risk of infection. Ascorbic acid (vitamin C) is an effective way to increase urine acidity, which helps decrease the chance of infection.
- Watch for the signs and symptoms listed in the Description section.
- Avoid substances that might cause irritation to the bladder including coffee and tea, alcoholic beverages, and tobacco products.
- Void (urinate) often.

OTHER MEASURES

- The physician will order blood and urine tests if the signs and symptoms of bladder irritation develop.
- Avoid coarse, fibrous foods.

CONSULT PHYSICIAN OR NURSE IF:

- You develop any of the signs or symptoms listed in the Description section.

——— BLEEDING (Thrombocytopenia) ———

DESCRIPTION

Radiation affects the cancerous and the normal cells in the body area receiving treatment. The platelet cells in your bone marrow divide quickly, and many may be injured by radiation treatment. Platelet cells are necessary for normal blood clotting. When your platelet count is low, you will have a tendency to bleed longer than you normally would. The nurse or physician will tell you if your platelet count is low.

DURATION

Decreased platelet count is temporary. Your bone marrow will replenish the platelet cells usually within 2 weeks. Your treatment will be postponed until your platelet count is within a normal range for you.

SELF-CARE MEASURES

- Watch for unexplained bruises (especially on the legs and feet).
- Be careful not to bump or cut yourself. If you start to bleed, apply pressure over the area with a bandage or clean piece of linen. Also, apply ice wrapped in a plastic bag over the area once the initial bleeding has stopped.
- Use an electric razor to avoid cuts.
- Brush your teeth gently with a soft brush or with your fingers.
- Do not take any type of injection unless absolutely necessary. Be sure the nurse or physician giving you an injection knows that your platelet count is low.
- If you must have blood drawn or be given an intravenous injection, put extra pressure on the needle site (5 minutes) to control bleeding after the needle is removed.
- Do not use any aspirin or products that contain aspirin. Check the labels of all drugs you are taking for salicylic acid. This ingredient is to be avoided. Use acetaminophen products. If you are not sure about a drug, ask your physician, nurse, or pharmacist whether you should use the drug while your platelet count is low.

- Avoid blowing your nose too hard or coughing too harshly.
- Take prescribed steroid medications with milk, food, or an antacid.
- Avoid use of alcohol.
- Avoid use of tampons.

OTHER MEASURES

- It may be necessary to give you a platelet transfusion if your platelet count is very low and you are having bleeding problems.
- Frequent blood tests will be necessary to monitor your platelet count.

CONSULT PHYSICIAN OR NURSE IF:

- You vomit or cough up blood, or there is blood in your stools (which might appear red or black and tarry) or in your urine.
- You experience coughing, vomiting, or tend to be constipated. Your physician will prescribe drugs for these conditions. A cough syrup is usually prescribed for your coughing. See Constipation in Chapter Two and Nausea and Vomiting in this chapter for self-care measures used for constipation and vomiting. Both of these symptoms are to be avoided to prevent bleeding of irritated tissues.

DIARRHEA

DESCRIPTION

Radiation treatment affects the cancer cells and the normal cells in the body area receiving treatment. The cells lining your mouth, stomach, and intestines divide rapidly, and if injured by radiation, may cause you to have diarrhea and may increase flatus (gas) and cramping. Severity of the diarrhea varies from person to person. The number of bowel movements may increase and your stools may be very soft or liquid.

DURATION

Diarrhea caused by radiation is temporary and self-limiting (sometimes stopping by itself). The cells lining the stomach and intestines will renew themselves. The diarrhea will stop when the treatment is completed.

SELF-CARE MEASURES

- Ask your physician to prescribe a drug (e.g., paregoric, Lomotil) to control the diarrhea. Kaopectate may not be effective for some people.
- Drink plenty of fluid that is at room temperature. Drink at least 3 quarts of liquid daily. Drinking more fluid does not cause more diarrhea, as some people think. You need the extra fluid to replace the fluid you are losing. Avoid extremely hot or cold fluids because these might increase bowel activity.
- Drink a liquid diet if the diarrhea becomes severe. Mild liquids such as fruit ades (e.g., Kool-Aid, Gatorade, liquid Jell-O) and peach or apricot nectar are usually well tolerated.
- Avoid food that contains roughage and bulk. Do not eat bran, whole-grain cereals skins and seeds, beans

and legumes, dried fruits, nuts, raw fruits, and vegetables.
- Avoid alcoholic beverages and tobacco products.
- Avoid drinking beverages while eating food. Drink liquids 30 minutes to 1 hour after the meal and between meals. Avoid foods and drinks that can produce gas or cause cramps such as beer, chewing gum, beans, cabbage, and sweets. Do not skip meals. Also avoid fatty, greasy, and spicy foods. Allow carbonated beverages to lose their fizz before drinking them. Avoid caffeinated beverages (e.g., coffee, tea, and colas).
- Eat foods high in potassium if the physician or nurse tells you that your potassium level is low. Examples are bananas, apricots without the skin, peach nectar, baked potatoes without the skin, broccoli, asparagus, meat, milk, saltwater fish, and mushrooms.
- Eat cottage cheese, applesauce, rice, and bananas instead of your regular meals for several days until the diarrhea decreases. Then gradually add food low in roughage and bulk such as mashed potatoes and dry toast. This diet is useful for severe diarrhea which happens infrequently.
- Keep an estimate of the number of stools (bowel movements) you have each day to guard against possible dehydration. The signs and symptoms of dehydration are dryness of your skin and mouth, decreased urine volume, sunken eyes, and marked fatigue.
- Apply over-the-counter ointment that contains lidocaine if your anal area is sore. For example, a layer of Desitin or A and D Ointment applied around the anal area can soothe irritation. Clean the area with warm water very gently but thoroughly after each bowel movement; then pat the area dry before applying the soothing lotions.

CONSULT PHYSICIAN OR NURSE IF:

• Your diarrhea becomes severe (more than four stools, liquid or formed, in a day) and the prescription drugs (e.g., paregoric) or over-the-counter drugs (e.g., Pepto-Bismol) are not effective. Other drugs, such as Lomotil or Immodium, can be prescribed.

ALSO SEE:

• Nausea and Vomiting, pages 167 to 170.
• Appetite, Decreased (Anorexia), pages 146 to 150.

———— EAR INFLAMMATION ————
(Otitis Media)

DESCRIPTION

Ear inflammation may result from radiation to the ear area. Symptoms include tinnitus (ringing in the ears), earache, and a feeling of fullness caused by a clogged eustachian tube.

DURATION

Symptoms subside with the completion of radiation treatment.

CONSULT PHYSICIAN OR NURSE IF:

• You notice any of these symptoms.

——— EYE INFLAMMATION ———
(Conjunctivitis)

DESCRIPTION

Inflammation of the eye may be a side effect of radiation to the eye. You may have symptoms of "bloodshot" eyes or burning eyes if the eye is directly irradiated.

DURATION

Mild episodes of inflammation of the eye will subside once radiation treatments are completed.

SELF-CARE MEASURES

- Avoid rubbing your eyes.
- Apply cool compresses to the eyes for 15 minutes three or four times a day.
- Wear sunglasses to lessen glare.

CONSULT PHYSICIAN OR NURSE IF:

- Any of the signs or symptoms occur.

——— HAIR THINNING ———
OR LOSS (Alopecia)

DESCRIPTION

You may lose some or all of your hair in the area being treated by radiation. Hair may fall out painlessly during grooming within 2 to 3 weeks after the start of treatment.

DURATION

Usually your hair will grow back after you have finished treatments, but if the dose of radiation is high, hair loss may be permanent. Regrowth usually occurs in 2 to 3 months, but the new hair may be of a different color and texture.

SELF-CARE MEASURES

- Keep your hair clean; wash it gently with a pH-balanced shampoo (e.g., Redken, Nexus).
- Use cream rinse and a soft-bristle brush to remove tangles.
- Avoid bleaching, teasing, rollers, permanents, and hair sprays, since they make the hair brittle, causing it to fall out faster during treatment.
- Cut hair to a short length and style to cover thinning spots.
- Buy wigs, scarves, and false eyelashes if you wish. They are tax-deductible medical expenses and may also be covered by your insurance. The head should not be covered with a wig all the time, but occasionally with a cotton scarf that allows the scalp to ''breathe.''
- Talk to the nurse or your physician about any feelings or questions you have about your altered appearance.

CONSULT PHYSICIAN OR NURSE IF:

- Your symptoms distress you.

———— INFECTION (Leukopenia) ————

DESCRIPTION

The cancerous cells and the normal cells that multiply quickly in the body site that receives the treatment will be injured by radiation. The white blood cells in your bone marrow may be injured and make you more susceptible to infections, but even if your white cell count is low, you may not get an infection. The signs and symptoms of an infection are sore throat, cough, and nasal congestion; burning when urinating; shaking chills; burning (pain) at the anus; pain, redness, swelling, and warmth at the site of injury to the skin; and fever. Eye or ear drainage can be a sign of infection.

DURATION

Low white blood cell production is a temporary side effect of treatment. Your body will replenish the white blood cells usually within 4 to 10 days. Your radiation treatment may be postponed until your white blood cell count is within a normal range for you.

SELF-CARE MEASURES

- Stay away from people with colds. Stay away from crowds. Avoid going to church, shopping, or movies at busy times, and so on. Your physician will tell you if these precautions are necessary.
- Take your temperature every 4 hours while awake if you have any signs of an infection. If you do not have a thermometer, buy one and ask the nurse to show you how to use it.
- Use antiseptic mouthwashes (e.g., Scope, Cepacol) daily, and have any dental problems taken care of to prevent possible infection.

- If you have an infection, drink 2 to 3 quarts of fluids a day; if you have a heart or kidney condition, ask the nurse or physician about this self-care measure.
- Perform excellent hygiene daily. Wash your hands before eating and after using the bathroom.
- Rest during the day if you become tired.
- Always wear shoes to prevent cuts on your feet.
- Protect your hands from cuts and burns. You can wear gloves while working in the garden, or wear rubber gloves while doing dishes.
- If you do get cut, wash the cut promptly with soap and water, and bandage it, if necessary.
- Avoid getting sunburned. Wear sunscreen (PABA #15 for maximum protection) and avoid being in the sun whenever possible.
- Do not take any vaccinations unless they have been approved by your physician. Avoid contact with adults and children who have recently been vaccinated against mumps, measles, polio, or smallpox. Avoid contact with anyone who has any of these conditions as well.
- Use a cuticle cream remover rather than cutting nail cuticles.
- Use a deodorant rather than an antiperspirant, which blocks sweat glands and may promote infection.
- Women should use sanitary napkins rather than tampons to reduce risk of infection.
- Use an electric razor to avoid breaks in the skin.
- Avoid rectal temperature taking and use of rectal suppositories.

OTHER MEASURES

- Frequent blood tests will be necessary to monitor the number of your white blood cells and the presence of an infection.

CONSULT PHYSICIAN OR NURSE IF:

- You experience any of the signs or symptoms of an infection.
- Your oral temperature goes above 101.5°F (38.6°C), or you experience shaking chills.

——— MOUTH PROBLEMS ———

Dry Mouth

DESCRIPTION

Radiation to your head and neck lessens the amount of saliva that your mouth membranes produce and causes a thickening of the saliva.

DURATION

Decreased saliva production begins 7 to 10 days after the start of therapy, reaches its peak within 2 to 3 weeks, and may persist weeks to months after the radiation treatment is completed.

SELF-CARE MEASURES

- Drink liquids often. Drink at least 3 quarts of fluid each day. Be sure to have liquids available to you. Keep liquids handy at your bedside and use a humidifier during the night. Carry a plastic bottle with you.
- Avoid breathing through your mouth.
- Inspect your mouth every morning for white patches.

- Suck on sugar-free hard candy or popsicles, or chew sugar-free gum. This may help to stimulate saliva production. Since tooth decay is a major problem, particularly for patients receiving radiation therapy to the head and neck area, the use of sugar-free products is best.
- Suck on ice chips or ice cubes that you've made from a beverage.
- Frequent cleansing of the mouth and teeth is necessary. Cleanse teeth with a soft-bristle toothbrush every 2 hours. Do not use commercial mouthwashes because they usually contain alcohol, which has a drying effect on the tissues lining the mouth. Make your own mouthwash by mixing 1 quart of warm water with 1 teaspoon of baking soda and ½ teaspoon of salt.
- Ask your physician or dentist about a fluoride mouthwash or artificial saliva.
- Eat soft, bland foods, especially cool or cold foods with a high liquid content, such as ice cream, popsicles, puddings, watermelon, and seedless grapes. Solid foods can be made easier to swallow by adding gravies, sauces, melted butter, broths, mayonnaise, yogurt, or salad dressing. Dunking bread and other baked foods in milk, tea, or coffee will make them easier to swallow.
- Avoid tobacco and alcohol.
- If you find solid foods too difficult to swallow, you should try a pureed diet or a full liquid diet with fruit ades or nectars. Since it may be difficult for you to eat enough during this time, adding a liquid high-protein supplement (examples of these are provided in the Nutrition Supplement of this book) to your diet will help ensure that you are getting enough protein and calories.

- Sip beverages between bites of food during meals.
- Avoid hot, spicy, or acidic foods.
- Artificial saliva can be purchased commercially* or prepared by your pharmacist.† Your dentist, nurse, or physician will advise you on its use. These products are not to be used if there are any sores in the mouth.

CONSULT PHYSICIAN OR NURSE IF:

- You observe creamy patches or streaks on the mucous lining of your mouth.

ALSO SEE:

- Appetite, Decreased (Anorexia), pages 146 to 150.

Mucositis

DESCRIPTION

Radiation to your head and neck may injure the mucosa, the lining in your mouth or digestive tract (esophagus). The signs of mucositis are extremely im-

---

*Zero-Lube, 1st Texas Pharmaceutical, Inc., 14335 Gillis Road, P.O. Drawer 400009, Dallas, TX 72450; Saliva-Aid, Copley Pharmaceutical, Inc., 398 West Second St., Boston, MA 02127; MVP Sports Gum, Amural Products, Naperville, IL 60540.

†The following formula for artificial saliva was developed at St. Jude Children's Research Hospital, Memphis, TN, by Raymond L. Braham, B.D.S., M.Sc. D., and Ronald D. Walker, D.D.S. It can be prepared by your pharmacist: carboxy methylcellulose 1 percent, 500 ml; glycerine, 200 ml; saline, 300 ml; cherry flavoring. The formula contains no preservatives and should be kept in the refrigerator. Fill a small plastic squeeze bottle for use during the day.

portant and should be evaluated promptly by your physician, because they may indicate that the tissues are reaching a temporary intolerance to treatment. This intolerance sometimes requires a rest from therapy for a few days to allow healing. Initially, there is inflammation of the mucous membranes; then a white or yellow glistening membrane covering may develop. The situation requires close observation by your physician (radiotherapist). Mucositis is a self-limiting condition that generally subsides 2 to 4 weeks after treatment.

SELF-CARE MEASURES

- Follow the suggestions listed in the sections on Dry Mouth and Stomatitis.

Stomatitis

DESCRIPTION

The cells lining your mouth and throat that grow quickly may be injured by radiation to your head and neck. Your mouth, gums, or throat may feel sore or different. You may see reddened areas in your mouth or gums that feel raw as if you accidentally bit the inside of your cheek while chewing.

DURATION

The degree and duration of the stomatitis depends on the depth of radiation penetration, the dose delivered, and the number of treatments. Mouth sores caused by radiation therapy are temporary. Your body's cellular lining in the mouth and throat regenerates. The mouth sores will heal when the treatment is completed, usually within 2 weeks.

SELF-CARE MEASURES

- Drink plenty of liquids to keep your mouth moist (e.g., lukewarm tea, Kool-Aid, and liquid Jell-O may be tolerated).
- Brush your teeth with a baby-soft toothbrush, or cleanse dentures after every meal to remove irritating food particles and to help prevent infection. Unwaxed dental floss should be used daily, but must be used gently. A water pick may also be used at a low setting.
- If you wear dentures, do not use gumlike grips. If your dentures do not fit well, have them adjusted by your dentist. Do not wear dentures, retainers, or partial plates if your mouth is sore. Wait until after radiation treatment is completed before having your dentures refitted.
- Be sure to gargle with your special mouthwash if it has been prescribed (e.g., Xylocaine 2% Viscous, Orabase, Dyclone). These mouthwashes contain medicine that helps ease the discomfort of mouth sores and promotes healing. They do not contain alcohol, which is irritating and drying to the mouth. Gargle 15 to 20 minutes before meals to help you feel more comfortable. If your gums are bleeding, do not use a toothbrush. Clean your teeth with a piece of moistened gauze or toothettes.
- Another recommended mouthwash recipe that has been helpful is 3½ ounces of Maalox and 1 ounce of Xylocaine 2% Viscous, plus the contents of a 25-milligram capsule of diphenhydramine hydrochloride (Benadryl). Shake well, use as a swish, and swallow or swish and spit. Repeat every 4 hours as needed. The solution should be kept in the refrigerator for an increased analgesic effect.

- Avoid very hot or very cold food since it may be irritating.
- Rinse your mouth frequently (at least every 4 hours).
- Make your own nonirritating mouthwash by mixing 1 teaspoon of baking soda with 1 quart of warm water. Keep the rinse in your mouth about 1 minute. Avoid commercial mouthwashes, as many contain salt and alcohol. Glycerine and lemon juice should never be used, since they cause the tissues of your mouth to become dry and irritated.
- Apply Blistex, cocoa butter, or baby oil to your lips to keep them moist.
- Eat bland and cool, soft foods such as custards, Jell-O, yogurt, soups, and eggs. Avoid foods such as oranges, tomatoes, lemons, limes, raw vegetables, or heavily spiced foods since they may irritate your mouth. Foods spiced with pepper, chili powder, and nutmeg may bother the mouth more than do foods spiced with cinnamon, garlic, or oregano. A peeled, grated fresh apple is easier to eat than a whole apple. Sucking on hard candies or popsicles may be soothing.
- Tylenol with codeine elixir can be swished in your mouth or swallowed for systemic and local relief. Keep in mind that the codeine can make you sleepy.
- Chew Aspergum, which can be purchased over the counter. Check with your nurse or physician first, since Aspergum may cause prolonged bleeding.
- Check your mouth and gums at least three times a day for any sores.
- Examine the oral cavity by removing all dental appliances. Use a good source of light, a glove or gauze, and a tongue blade to move the tongue and lips out of the way so you can see all surfaces. Use a dental mirror to see further back in the throat.

- If your home is heated with dry heat, a humidifier or a steam kettle in the bedroom may help.
- Drink soft food from a cup or through a straw if you are having trouble eating with a fork or spoon.
- Add sauces and gravies to solid foods, or puree or liquefy foods if you have decreased saliva or difficulty in swallowing.
- Avoid tobacco, snuff, and alcohol.
- Talk with your physician or nurse in the radiation department before having dental work done. Make sure your dentist knows you are receiving radiation.
- Ask your dentist about the daily use of fluoride gel to help prevent severe tooth decay that can develop when the flow of saliva is reduced.

——— NAUSEA AND VOMITING ———

DESCRIPTION

Radiation treatment may cause slight nausea or severe episodes of vomiting, depending on the body area being treated. It could result from stimulation of the nausea centers in your brain or irritation of your digestive tract lining by the radiation. Nausea is more likely to occur with radiation to the abdominal or pelvic areas, or if you receive chemotherapy with radiation therapy.

DURATION

Nausea generally begins 4 to 6 hours after the treatment has begun, lasts a few hours, and then disappears. Nausea and vomiting usually permanently disappear within 1 week after you complete your treatment.

SELF-CARE MEASURES

- Ask for an antinausea pill, suppository, or shot 30 to 60 minutes before each treatment, and take the pill or suppository every 4 hours if you need it. Marijuana may be prescribed by the physician in some states.
- Take an antacid (e.g., Maalox) after taking the antinausea medicine. Avoid unnecessary movement.
- Eat small snacks (five to six times a day). Sweet or salty foods may be tolerated.
- Rest after meals. Activity can aggravate the nausea. If you recline after meals, make sure your head is 4 inches higher than your feet.
- Drink liquids frequently (but not with meals) if you are able to drink. It is essential that the fluids you drink contain salt, when vomiting is severe or prolonged, to make up for the body's loss of water and salt. Broth and Gatorade, for example, contain salt.
- Avoid hot foods. Their odors sometimes make nausea worse. Try cold meat and fruit plates with cottage cheese, and small sandwiches of bland food.
- Take a pain pill, if you are in pain, before the pain becomes more severe.
- Eating saltine crackers when you feel nauseated may prevent dry heaves. Also eat the crackers before you take the pain medication if you already feel queasy, as they will reduce the nausea you may experience after taking the pain medicine.
- Only drink fluids for several hours after each treatment. It may be helpful to eat a light snack at least 1 to 2 hours before the treatment since for several hours after each treatment you should only drink fluids.

- When you are nauseated, try to distract yourself with activities you particularly enjoy, for example, listening to music, sleeping, talking about pleasant things; try self-hypnosis or slow mouth breathing.
- Avoid greasy foods because they take longer to leave the stomach; carbohydrate-containing foods leave the stomach more quickly. The volume of food in the stomach can be reduced by avoiding liquids at mealtimes and by drinking them 1 hour before or after eating.
- Keep track of how much fluid you drink and how much you urinate to assess possible dehydration. The signs and symptoms of dehydration are dryness of skin and mouth, decreased urine volume, and excessive fatigue.
- Talk with your physician about scheduling the treatment later in the day. The effects of nausea and vomiting may cause you to miss the evening meal, but you may regain some appetite by morning. Keep track of your sickness patterns, recording the onset and duration. By knowing your particular pattern of sickness you can determine better when to apply the self-care measures or what treatment time would be best for you.
- Clean your mouth well before meals and brush your teeth soon after eating.
- Rinse your mouth with a mouthwash or with a solution of warm water and lemon juice after vomiting.
- Avoid doing your own cooking if the odor nauseates you. Sit in another room or take a walk while the food is being cooked.
- Eat slowly so that only small amounts of food enter your stomach at one time.
- Chew your food well so you can digest it more easily.

- Do not force yourself to eat more than you can possibly manage.
- Get fresh air by sitting near an open window or outdoors.
- Salty food, pretzels, and crackers may decrease nausea.

CONSULT PHYSICIAN OR NURSE IF:

- You have been vomiting and have not been able to keep anything down for 24 hours and/or you are noticing the signs and symptoms of dehydration.
- You are bloated, are in pain, or have a swollen stomach before an episode of vomiting, especially if these symptoms are relieved by vomiting.

ALSO SEE:

- Appetite, Decreased (Anorexia), pages 146 to 150.

——— RADIATION ———
LHERMITTE'S SIGN

DESCRIPTION

Radiation therapy to the cervical spinal cord can produce a transient syndrome called electrical parasthenia that affects arms and legs. The symptoms include numbness and tingling.

DURATION

Numbness and tingling usually occur 1 to 2 months after completion of radiation treatment, and may last several months.

SELF-CARE MEASURES

- Protect the affected limb from injury while you are experiencing these symptoms. Avoid potentially injurious activities and exposure to extreme heat or cold.

CONSULT PHYSICIAN OR NURSE IF:

- You experience progressive weakness and numbness of the arms or legs.

——— RADIATION PNEUMONITIS ———

DESCRIPTION

If more than 25 percent of the lung tissue is exposed to radiation, you may experience fever, mild shortness of breath, dry cough, and weakness because the normal lung tissue is reacting to the treatment.

DURATION

Radiation pneumonitis can occur 1 to 3 months or even 1 year after radiation therapy is completed, and can be either temporary or permanent.

SELF-CARE MEASURES

- Pace your activities so that you do not become too short of breath. To decrease the frequency of a dry, hacking, persistent cough, humidify the air with a cold-water vaporizer, a pan of water on a source of heat, or a humidifier as part of the central heating system.
- Drink warm fluids or suck on a cough drop or throat lozenge when the cough becomes persistent.

- Force fluids (3 quarts daily) unless restricted for other illnesses.

CONSULT PHYSICIAN OR NURSE IF:

- You become short of breath, develop a fever, or develop a dry cough.

——— RADIATION SYNDROME ———

DESCRIPTION

Radiation treatment may cause you to experience some generalized symptoms not specifically related to the radiated body area. These signs and symptoms may include fatigue, malaise (generally feeling poorly), headache, anorexia, diarrhea, nausea, and vomiting. The symptoms are related to the volume of tissue radiated and the daily dose of radiation you receive. The breakdown products from rapid tumor cell destruction may cause the radiation syndrome. The syndrome occurs mainly in individuals who receive radiation in the chest and upper or lower abdominal regions.

DURATION

You may experience the symptoms as long as you are receiving the current dosage of radiation. However, adjustments in your radiation treatment can be made so that the symptoms lessen.

SELF-CARE MEASURES

- For fatigue and malaise, refer to the Anemia section.
- For anorexia, see Appetite, Decreased (Anorexia).

- For diarrhea, nausea, and vomiting, see the so-named sections.

CONSULT PHYSICIAN OR NURSE IF:

- You develop the symptoms of radiation syndrome.

—— SEXUAL DYSFUNCTION ——
Impotence

DESCRIPTION

In men, an inability may develop to gain or maintain erection. It may be temporary or permanent, depending on the degree of injury to the cells. Men who are receiving high-dose radiation (7,000 rads) to the prostate gland are at risk.

DURATION

The long-term effect of radiation therapy on normal sexual function should be discussed with your physician before treatment begins. Twenty-five percent of men at risk (see above) will experience nerve impotence 1 to 2 years after treatment.

SELF-CARE MEASURES

- Engage in other satisfying ways of expressing affection while the side effects of treatment are occurring.
- Since you can still father children, you or your partner must use a birth-control method.

CONSULT PHYSICIAN OR NURSE IF:

• You develop impotence.

ALSO SEE:

• Sexual Dysfunction, Sterility, pages 176 to 178.

Menstrual Changes

DESCRIPTION

Radiation treatment to the pelvic area may change your menstrual cycle. You may stop menstruating or note a change in the length of your periods. Your normal amount of flow may be changed; spotting between menstruation may occur. Symptoms of menopause appear in women who stop menstruating while receiving radiation.

DURATION

Menstrual changes will continue for the duration of your treatment. Radiation of the ovaries can cause temporary or permanent cessation of ovulation.

SELF-CARE MEASURES

• Be prepared for menstrual changes by carrying a supply of feminine hygiene products.
• Contraception should be used due to the adverse effects of radiation therapy on the fetus.

CONSULT PHYSICIAN OR NURSE IF:

- You start spotting during your menstrual cycle. The spotting may be from other causes besides radiation.

ALSO SEE:

- Sexual Dysfunction, Sterility, pages 176 to 178.

Painful Intercourse

DESCRIPTION

Women who receive radiation to the pelvic area experience pain during intercourse from insufficient lubrication of the vagina due to lowered levels of estrogen (female hormone).

DURATION

Decreased lubrication caused by radiation treatment may or may not be temporary, depending on the degree of damage to the lubricating glands. Shortening of the vagina can be progressive unless self-care measures are done.

SELF-CARE MEASURES

For lubrication:

- Apply over-the-counter lubricants such as K-Y Jelly, Slippery Stuff, or Albane.
- Avoid products like petroleum jelly or other ointments that have an oil base. The lotions you use must be water-soluble.

For shortening of the vagina:

- Insert the dilators provided by your physician at least three times a week.
- Continue sexual intercourse as tolerable by comfort and physical limitation to prevent or to minimize the degree of vaginal stenosis that may occur several weeks or months after the course of treatment has ended. Ideally, intercourse would be at least three times a week during radiation treatment. Check with your radiotherapist regarding intercourse during treatment.
- Use different positions during intercourse, especially sitting or lying on top of your partner, enabling you to move in ways that are pleasurable rather than painful.

CONSULT PHYSICIAN OR NURSE IF:

- Intercourse continues to be painful.

Sterility

DESCRIPTION

Gonad function in men and women may be affected by radiation treatment to the pelvic area. There may be a transient decrease in the number of sperm. Ovulation may not occur during radiation therapy.

DURATION

In women, when the ovaries are exposed to radiation, temporary or permanent sterility may occur depending on the radiation dose, the volume of tissues radiated, and the time period the ovaries are exposed to radiation.

The amount of radiation required to produce sterility depends on the woman's age at the time she receives radiation treatment. The younger the woman, the greater will be the number of ova in the ovaries; therefore, a greater amount of radiation will be required before sterility occurs. If permanent sterility occurs, the menstrual cycle will be altered initially and then stop altogether. If sterility is temporary, your normal menstrual pattern may not resume for 6 months to 1 year after treatment. Because the ova may have been exposed to radiation, genetic changes may be present.

In men, sterility may occur during radiation treatment without permanent loss of potency. Potency, the ability to get or maintain an erection, remains. Destruction of sperm will not affect sexual drive. Chromosomal damage can occur in radiated sperm. Normal sperm count and viability may be reestablished once radiation treatment is completed; this factor depends on the amount of radiation to the testes. Permanent sterility usually occurs with more than 500 rads to the testes.

SELF-CARE MEASURES

- Talk with your physician or nurse about the most effective method of birth control for you, given the adverse effects radiation can have on fetal development.
- Wait 2 years after treatment before trying to conceive.

OTHER MEASURES

- In men, ask your physician about freezing some of your sperm for future use before beginning radiation therapy.

- In women, ask your physician about oophoropexy, a surgical tucking away of the ovaries out of the potential treatment field, which may preserve fertility. Your surgeon and radiation oncologist will need to talk to each other about this situation before radiation therapy begins.

CONSULT PHYSICIAN OR NURSE IF:

- You are having any sexual dysfunction.

———— SKIN PROBLEMS ————

DESCRIPTION

Sometimes the skin in the radiation treatment area may begin to look red, irritated (peeling), tanned, or sunburned.

DURATION

The skin reaction usually occurs during your second week of treatment, increases until about 7 days after your final radiation treatment, and then subsides, usually 2 to 4 weeks after treatment. The skin reactions that look dry (peeling) are a result of temporary damage to the sweat and sebaceous glands.

SELF-CARE MEASURES

- Do not use heating lamps, ice packs, hot-water bottles, or anything besides warm (never hot) water on your skin, because your ability to tolerate heat or cold without skin damage is lowered.

- Use mild soaps while bathing. Avoid scrubbing or vigorous wiping with a towel. Be careful not to wash off any of the skin marks. If the skin marks come off, do not attempt to redraw them. When you arrive for your next treatment, tell the technician they came off. Many radiation therapy departments use a small tattoo to demarcate the area to be treated. If this is the case, the tattoo will not wash off.
- Be careful of the radiated area since it is more vulnerable to infection and breakdown.
- Do not use adhesive tape on skin in treated areas.
- During treatment, wear shirts, blouses, or neck scarves that are soft and have soft collars (no starch). Clothing that rubs the treated area should be avoided. Women should not wear tight straps, brassieres, girdles, corsets, or belts. Men should not wear tight collars, belts, or trousers. Fabric of 100 percent cotton is usually recommended for clothing in contact with the area. Two weeks after radiation therapy is completed, if the skin is fully healed, a brassiere can be worn. However, it should be worn only part of the day and then removed. Upon removing the brassiere, check to see if there are areas of irritation. If there are, do not wear the brassiere without protecting that portion of your skin with padding. Frequently, a cotton shirt worn under the brassiere provides greater comfort. After a mastectomy that is followed by radiation therapy a prosthetic brassiere—which is usually heavier than a regular brassiere—should not be worn for at least 6 weeks after the final radiation treatment.
- Use only an electric razor and do not shave within the treated areas. The therapy will lessen hair growth in the treated areas. Do not use a preshave or aftershave lotion.

- Do not apply any lotion, underarm deodorant, powder, or cream to the treated skin since these may cause aggravation of the irritated area, and they may contain metal bases that could change the absorption of radiation. Application (with your physician's approval) of bland ointments that are water-soluble, such as vitamins A and D and glycerine, Aquaphor, lanolin, Lubriderm, and baby oil, will counteract the dryness and itching. Hydrocortisone creams will assist in reduction of inflammation and must be prescribed by your physician since they constrict (decrease) blood flow to the skin and should not be used when your skin reaction is wet and draining.
- Do not scratch the treated skin. If the skin in the treated area begins to itch or cause discomfort, discuss the problem with your physician.
- While undergoing treatment, do not expose the treated area to strong sunlight, cold temperature, winds or rain. (Sun exposure is the most intense from 11 A.M. to 2 P.M.; sunscreen rated 15 completely blocks the sun's rays.) Protect the area of skin being treated by clothing (e.g., long-sleeved cotton shirts, hats). In winter weather, warm clothing is important. After treatment is completed, very strong sunlight should be avoided or enjoyed in limited doses. Use of sunscreens is recommended.
- Provide thorough skin care to areas of high risk for breakdown. These are areas where there are folds of the skin, particularly in the groin, between the legs, under the arms, under the breasts, buttocks, and behind the ears.
- To absorb moisture in skin-fold areas where two skin surfaces touch, use cornstarch, which is also an effective anti-itching agent. Use the cornstarch only when your skin reaction to treatment is dry, not wet and draining.

- Check the skin at the entry site of the radiation beam as well as the skin at the exit site (the other side of your body) every other day. Signs and symptoms of infection should be carefully watched. The inflammatory response may be masked by redness and swelling caused by radiation.

CONSULT PHYSICIAN OR NURSE IF:

- The skin at the radiation site becomes moist or sticky, if it blisters, or if it breaks.

——— SWALLOWING DIFFICULTY ———
(Esophagitis)

DESCRIPTION

Esophagitis, an inflammation of the lining of the esophagus, which is the tube that goes from your throat to your stomach, may be a side effect of radiation therapy to the head, neck, and upper chest area. You may have temporary discomfort because of pain, swelling, or dryness of the throat, or more severe problems such as dehydration.

DURATION

Difficulty in swallowing may lessen while you are still receiving your radiation treatment. Usually the symptom stops 2 to 4 weeks after completion of your treatment.

SELF-CARE MEASURES

- Gargle and swallow an analgesic (pain-relieving) solution such as liquid Xylocaine before meals. Another solution may be made by mixing 1 tablespoon of sour cream with 1 tablespoon of liquid Tylenol. Systemic analgesics (which go to the whole body) such as Tylenol or codeine may also be needed to relieve pain.

- Eat frequent small meals (six per day). Solid foods should be soft and cooked until tender. They should be cut into bite-sized pieces and moistened with liberal amounts of gravies, mayonnaise, salad dressing, sauces, sour cream, or yogurt.
- Choose single-textured foods (such as oatmeal) instead of combination foods (such as stew) since similar textures will be easier to swallow.
- Avoid hard or dry foods such as crackers, nuts, seeds, popcorn, potato chips, pretzels, and raw vegetables.
- Avoid a liquid diet because liquids can accidentally go down your windpipe and cause you to gag or choke. Beverages of a thick, milkshakelike consistency are safer than thin liquids.
- Eat a liquid high-protein diet supplement thickened with ice cream to ensure an adequate protein and calorie intake. Custard, fortified Jell-O, and pudding are easy to swallow and are good protein and calorie supplements.
- Put cold (not iced) compresses on your throat for 30 minutes before eating.
- Stimulate swallowing and increase saliva by sucking on popsicles, lollipops, small bits of crushed ice, or a piece of cheesecloth soaked in ice water or juice. If increasing saliva is the problem, remember that sour foods increase saliva and sweet foods decrease it.
- Experiment with food temperature. Generally, foods served at room temperature, rather than very cold or very hot, can be more comfortably swallowed.

- Include applesauce, cold liquids, cooked cereals, strained cream soup, custard, soft-cooked eggs, plain ice cream, gelatin, milkshakes, mashed potatoes, pudding, or sherbet in your diet.
- Avoid spices such as pepper, chili powder, nutmeg, curry, and cloves.
- If swallowing becomes extremely difficult, it may be necessary to tilt the head upward so the food flows to the back of the throat before swallowing.
- Chew Aspergum 30 minutes before eating.
- Weigh yourself every other day.

CONSULT PHYSICIAN OR NURSE IF:

- Your difficulty in swallowing becomes suddenly worse.
- You begin to lose weight because you are not eating.

——————TASTE AND SMELL CHANGES——————

DESCRIPTION

Radiation treatment to the head and neck areas may change your sense of taste or smell or both. Foods may taste bitter or rancid, and you may have aversions to certain foods. Taste buds are special tissues that detect the substances in foods that are responsible for the different tastes. The four basic tastes are sweet, sour, bitter, and sharp. The ability to tell the difference between tastes varies depending on the intensity of the chemical substance in the food and the condition of the taste buds. The tongue's lining and taste buds are changed by radiation.

DURATION

After healing, your taste may return partially or completely to its former sensitivity (discrimination). It may be 3 to 6 months after completion of therapy before your sense of taste is normal again.

SELF-CARE MEASURES

- Since taste changes commonly include aversion to several of the most popular protein foods, such as meat, poultry, fish, and eggs, look for other, more palatable foods that are also good sources of protein, such as milk, ice cream, bland cheese, cottage cheese, and peanut butter. A vegetarian or Chinese cookbook can provide useful, nonmeat, high-protein recipes.
- Use plastic rather than metal utensils to decrease the bitter taste of foods.
- Try to eat warmed cured meats such as ham, bacon, sausage, and corned beef; you may want to marinate meats in soy sauce if you are not on a salt-restricted diet. Meats can be marinated in sweet fruit juices or sweet wines and cooked with fruit over them to improve the taste.
- Eat frequent small meals. It may be helpful to add a liquid high-protein diet supplement.
- Prepare foods that look and smell appetizing. Fresh fruits, gelatin salads, and lettuce are generally appealing.
- Seasonings, including lemon juice, mint, and basil, will help improve the taste and aroma of food. Experiment with different flavor extracts. Extra sugar can be used. Do not try to follow any particular rule in seasoning, but use your imagination and experi-

ment. Take additional precautions if dryness of the mouth, mucositis, or both occur.

- Continue to eat even though taste alterations are present. Food should be considered as important as the treatment. Without adequate protein and calories, the normal cells that are being destroyed will be unable to repair themselves.
- Ask your physician about prescribing a zinc supplement to your diet.
- Cold plates such as cottage cheese and fruit and chicken salad may be more appealing than hot foods.

CONSULT PHYSICIAN OR NURSE IF:

- Your food intake is reduced over time.
- You are losing more than 2 pounds per week.

ALSO SEE:

- Appetite, Decreased (Anorexia), pages 146 to 150.
- Mouth Problems, Dry Mouth, pages 161 to 163; Mucositis, pages 163 to 164; Stomatitis, pages 164 to 167.

——— TOOTH DECAY ———

DESCRIPTION

Because of the effects of radiation to your head on teeth and saliva, your teeth will be very susceptible to decay.

DURATION

The effects of radiation to your mouth and teeth may be permanent. Therefore, you may need to continue the self-care measures to prevent decay throughout your life.

SELF-CARE MEASURES

- Have a dentist examine your teeth before radiation treatment to determine which teeth, if any, are likely to be affected by radiation therapy or cause problems in the future. These teeth should be treated before radiation treatment while your ability to heal is not yet reduced. After the completion of therapy, visit your dentist every 6 months.
- Avoid foods and beverages high in sugar. Sugar-free candy and beverages are preferable.
- Clean your teeth and gums with a brush with soft, rounded bristles four times a day. Use a fluoride toothpaste and make sure the toothpaste has no rough grains in it.
- Floss twice a day because brushing alone does not clean between teeth.
- Use a disclosing solution or tablet (made of a harmless red vegetable dye) that will reveal, by red color, any plaque you failed to remove in brushing and flossing. Use the disclosing solution after you brush in the evening to show where you have failed to brush adequately.
- Rinse your mouth well (mix 1 quart of warm water with ½ teaspoon of salt and 1 teaspoon of baking soda). Use this solution after each brushing and periodically to refresh your mouth.
- Apply fluoride at least once a day, preferably after brushing. The dentist will instruct you on a method most suitable for your needs (fluoride rinse, fluoride gel, or fluoride tablets). The dentist can prescribe fluoride gel in small trays that fit over your teeth like an athlete's mouth guard. Fluoride mouthwashes may also be used.

- Do not use commercial mouthwashes, as they contain up to 28 percent alcohol, which may dry your gums. A dry mouth makes teeth more likely to stay unclean and, therefore, more prone to decay.
- Remove your dentures, retainers, or partials for a few hours each day and at night to relieve the pressure from these appliances. Have your dentist check to make sure your dentures fit properly before and after treatment.

CONSULT PHYSICIAN OR NURSE IF:

- You develop a toothache or a tooth is loose.

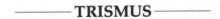

TRISMUS

DESCRIPTION

Radiation treatment to the chewing (masticating) muscles may result in their dysfunction, allowing for only a small opening of the mouth.

DURATION

Trismus is a late effect of radiation therapy, and may become progressive if corrective measures are not taken.

SELF-CARE MEASURES

- Use individually designed appliances to enable greater opening of the mouth.
- Do exercises prescribed by your physician to decrease the dysfunction of the chewing muscles.

CONSULT PHYSICIAN OR NURSE IF:

• You suddenly have difficulty opening your mouth.

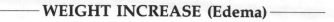

—————— WEIGHT INCREASE (Edema) ——————

DESCRIPTION

The lymph nodes that drain the fluid from your arms or legs may be injured by radiation therapy in combination with surgery, causing edema (puffy arms or legs). The problem occurs if lymph nodes were removed from the axilla or groin during surgery.

DURATION

The edema can occur during radiation treatment or after it is completed.

SELF-CARE MEASURES

• Avoid tight clothes that slow down circulation to the arms or legs. TED hose or Jobst stockings can be worn after asking your nurse or physician about their use.
• Avoid injury to the arms or legs, because with edema the injury is more likely to become infected. Be careful when caring for your nails, use an electric razor for shaving, and wear gloves for such potentially injurious activities as gardening. No blood specimens or blood pressure measures should be taken from an arm that has edema.

- Elevate the puffy arms or legs above heart level whenever possible. If the legs are affected, do not stand in one place for a long time. Do not cross your legs when sitting.

CONSULT PHYSICIAN OR NURSE IF:

- You experience a sudden or severe swelling in your arms or legs.

PART III

The Self-Care Behaviors Log and Patient Appointment Worksheet

THE SELF-CARE BEHAVIORS LOG

The Self-Care Behaviors Log is divided into two sections. The first section is where you will list the potential side effects of your chemotherapy or radiation therapy. These side effects would have been identified for you by your doctor and nurse when the treatment was explained to you. In this section you will write in the actions you have taken to prevent these potential side effects. Finally, you will write in the name of the person, including yourself, who suggested the actions to prevent the side effects.

The second section is where you will list any experienced side effect of your chemotherapy or radiation therapy. Circle the numbers (1 to 5) that correspond to the degree of severity and distress it is causing. Next, list any actions you took to alleviate the side effect and circle how effective the actions were on the effectiveness scale (1 to 5). Finally, write in the name of the person, including yourself, who suggested the actions to alleviate the side effects.

Potential Side Effects You Are Susceptible to Develop	Actions Taken to Prevent Side Effects		Sources of Suggestions for Actions
1. _____	a. _____ b. _____ c. _____ d. _____	date: ____ date: ____ date: ____ date: ____	a. _____ b. _____ c. _____ d. _____
2. _____	a. _____ b. _____ c. _____ d. _____	date: ____ date: ____ date: ____ date: ____	a. _____ b. _____ c. _____ d. _____
3. _____	a. _____ b. _____ c. _____ d. _____	date: ____ date: ____ date: ____ date: ____	a. _____ b. _____ c. _____ d. _____
4. _____	a. _____ b. _____ c. _____ d. _____	date: ____ date: ____ date: ____ date: ____	a. _____ b. _____ c. _____ d. _____

Potential Side Effects You Are Susceptible to Develop	Actions Taken to Prevent Side Effects		Sources of Suggestions for Actions
5. _____	a. _____	date: _____	a. _____
	b. _____	date: _____	b. _____
	c. _____	date: _____	c. _____
	d. _____	date: _____	d. _____
6. _____	a. _____	date: _____	a. _____
	b. _____	date: _____	b. _____
	c. _____	date: _____	c. _____
	d. _____	date: _____	d. _____
7. _____	a. _____	date: _____	a. _____
	b. _____	date: _____	b. _____
	c. _____	date: _____	c. _____
	d. _____	date: _____	d. _____
8. _____	a. _____	date: _____	a. _____
	b. _____	date: _____	b. _____
	c. _____	date: _____	c. _____
	d. _____	date: _____	d. _____

Experienced Side Effect(s) from Chemotherapy/Radiation Therapy

Experienced Side Effect(s) from Chemotherapy/Radiation Therapy	Actions Taken	Effectiveness of Actions	Sources of Suggestions for Actions

1. _____

a. Severity of side effect—i.e., how intense is it?

barely noticeable			most severe
1	2	3	4	5

Date of onset _____

b. Distress of side effect—i.e., how much does it bother you?

minor annoyance			extremely distressing
1	2	3	4	5

Actions Taken

a. _____
_____
_____
_____
_____
_____

Date: _____

b. _____
_____
_____
_____
_____

Effectiveness of Actions

Not Relieved at All			Completely Relieved
1	2	3	4	5

| 1 | 2 | 3 | 4 | 5 |

Sources of Suggestions for Actions

a. _____

b. _____

2. _____

a. Severity of side effect— i.e., how intense is it?

barely noticeable   **most severe**

1   2   3   4   5

a. _____   1   2   3   4   5   a. _____

Date of onset _____

Date: _____

b. Distress of side effect— i.e., how much does it bother you?

minor annoyance   **extremely distressing**

1   2   3   4   5

b. _____   1   2   3   4   5   b. _____

Date: _____

Experienced Side Effect(s) from Chemotherapy/Radiation Therapy	Actions Taken	Effectiveness of Actions	Sources of Suggestions for Actions

3. _____

a. Severity of side effect— i.e., how intense is it?

barely noticeable   **most severe**

1   2   3   4   5

Date of onset _____

b. Distress of side effect— i.e., how much does it bother you?

minor annoyance   **extremely distressing**

1   2   3   4   5

Actions Taken

a. _____
_____
_____
_____
_____
_____

Date: _____

b. _____
_____
_____
_____
_____

Effectiveness of Actions

Not Relieved at All   Completely Relieved

1   2   3   4   5

1   2   3   4   5

Sources of Suggestions for Actions

a. _____

b. _____

————PATIENT APPOINTMENT———— WORKSHEET

My next scheduled appointment is:

<u>DATE</u>
<u>TIME</u>
<u>COMMENTS</u>

Questions I will ask the doctor or nurse:

Things I must remember to tell the doctor or nurse:

Other things I must remember:

BIBLIOGRAPHY

Dodd, M. J. 1982a. Chemotherapy knowledge in patients with cancer: Assessment and informational interventions. *Oncology Nursing Forum* 9(3):39–44.

Dodd, M.J. 1982b. Assessing patient self-care for side effects of cancer chemotherapy. *Cancer Nursing* 5:447–451.

Dodd, M. J. 1983. Self-care for side effects of cancer chemotherapy: An assessment of nursing interventions. *Cancer Nursing* 6:63–67.

Dodd, M. J. 1984a. Measuring informational intervention for chemotherapy and self-care behavior. *Research in Nursing and Health* 7:43–50.

Dodd, M. J. 1984b. Patterns of self-care in cancer patients receiving radiation therapy. *Oncology Nursing Forum* 10(3):23–27.

Dodd, M.J. 1984c. Self-care for preventing side effects by breast cancer patients in chemotherapy. *Public Health Nursing* 1(4):202–209.

Dodd, M. J. 1987. Efficacy of proactive information on self-care in radiation therapy patients. *Heart and Lung* 16(5):538–544.

Dodd, M. J. 1988a. Patterns of self-care in patients with breast cancer. *Western Journal of Nursing* 10(1):7–24.

Dodd, M. J. 1988b. Efficacy of proactive information on self-care in chemotherapy patients. *Patient Education and Counseling* 11:215–225.

Dodd, M. J., and D. W. Mood. 1981. Chemotherapy: Retention and review of information. *Cancer Nursing* 4(4):311–318.

Free publications related to cancer and its treatment are available from either the American Cancer Society's local (county) unit or the National Cancer Institute's toll-free number (1-800-4-CANCER).

INDEX

Index

Ears *(continued)*
  see also Hearing loss
Edema, 7, 13, 15, 33, 44, 125–127,
  188–189
  see also Heart damage; Weight
  increase
Electrical parasthenia, 170–171
Electrocardiograms, 82
Elspar, 33
Esophagitis, 121, 181–183
Estrogen, 25
Etoposide [VP-16], 26–27
Eulexin, 29–30
Extrapyramidal symptoms, 99
Extravasation, 114–115
  cisplatin and, 16
  dacarbazine and, 19
  dactinomycin and, 20
  daunorubicin hydrochloride and,
  21
  doxorubicin hydrochloride and, 25
  mechlorethamine hydrochloride,
  37
  mitomycin and, 44
  streptozocin and, 49
  vinblastine sulfate and, 54
  vincristine sulfate and, 55
Eyes, 87, 157
  see also Visual disorders

F
  aminoglutethimide and, 6
  L-asparaginase and, 33
  floxuride and, 28
  fluorouracil and, 29
  hexamethylmelamine and, 31
  ifosfamide and, 32
  maytansine and, 36
  methotrexate and, 42
  vincristine sulfate and, 54
Feminization. *See* Sexual dysfunction

Fertility, 50, 109
Fever, 75–77
  L-asparaginase and, 33
  azacytidine and, 8
  bleomycin sulfate and, 9
  busulfan and, 10
  etoposide and, 26
  melphalan and, 39
  mercaptopurine and, 41
  mitoxantrone hydrochloride and,
  45
  thio-tepa and, 52
  see also Hot flashes; Infection
Fingernails, 105
Fluid retention. *See* Edema
Flulike syndrome, 18, 19, 47, 77–78
Fluoride, 186
Fluorouracil [5-FU], 28–29
Flutamide, 29–30
Food intolerance, 48, 74
Foxuride [FUDR], 27–28

G
Gastric ulcers. *See* Stomach irritation

H
Hair, 78–80
Hair loss, 157–158
  amsacrine and, 7
  belomycin sulfate and, 9
  cyclophosphamide and, 17
  dacarbazine and, 19
  dactinomycin and, 20
  daunorubicin hydrochloride and,
  22
  doxorubicin hydrochloride and, 24
  etoposide and, 26
  floxuride and, 27
  fluorouracil and, 29
  hexamethylmelamine and, 30
  ifosfamide and, 33

ABOUT THE AUTHOR

Marylin Dodd, R.N., Ph.D., is a professor in nursing at the University of California San Francisco School of Nursing. She has also worked as a nurse practitioner in private practice specializing in working with cancer patients and their families.